The A.N.G.E.L. Plan

A New Godly Eating Lifestyle

I cannot overemphasize the importance of morning devotions in *The A.N.G.E.L. Plan—A New Godly Eating Lifestyle©*.

ROSEMARY RYAN-DELP

ISBN 979-8-89043-184-4 (paperback)
ISBN 979-8-89043-185-1 (digital)

Christian Faith Publishing
832 Park Avenue
Meadville, PA 16335
www.christianfaithpublishing.com

Printed in the United States of America

To **Jesus Christ**; to my lifelong friend, **Janet McLeland**, who found freedom in *The A.N.G.E.L. Plan©* and lost fifty pounds and who painstakingly and freely edited my book; and **Brandon Delp**, my husband and partner, for his endless patience with my writing and editing this book. Priceless!

CONTENTS

---

[1] Chapter 13 can mean personal bankruptcy, and we just won't go there. With God, we are never bankrupt!

FOREWORD

Please allow me to introduce myself. My name is Rosemary Ryan-Delp, and I am a Christian. I believe in God the Father, Jesus Christ the Son and our Savior, the Holy Spirit of Jesus Christ, a Trinity who is all-loving, all-powerful, all-knowing. This book is written from that perspective.

I also believe in the inspiration and anointing of the Holy Spirit to help me write, proofread, edit and rewrite, and also to find the right editor, literary agent, and publisher. The Holy Spirit so *diligently* impressed me to write this book that I truly believe God wanted me to put *The A.N.G.E.L. Plan: A New Godly Eating Lifestyle*© into print so that it might help others as much as it has helped me!

CAUTION: AS BEFORE, ANY CHANGE IN EATING HABITS, PLEASE CHECK WITH YOUR PHYSICIAN BEFORE EMBRACING *THE A.N.G.E.L. PLAN: A NEW GODLY EATING LIFESTYLE*©!

I ask only that you allow yourself to **open your eyes to the possibili-ties and concepts incorporated in this book.** They have certainly changed my life and healed my body in so many miraculous ways! Enjoy the book!

PREFACE

God didn't say anywhere in His Word that people should count pounds or calories or fats or proteins or carbohydrates or grams or ounces or macros.

God did not say we are to completely abstain from food indefinitely.

God did not tell us to wear a certain pants size or dress size or to try to live up to other people's standards about what we wear or how we look on the outside.

It's what flows from our inside that counts! *Are you flowing God's love, or are you flowing pride or self-recrimination?*

What **GOD DID EMPHASIZE** is that we are **to fast and pray for,** among other things, **forgiveness of others and deliverance from temptation;** and we may be healed of so many things.

Jesus specifically told us that some demons *(diseases, overeating, alcoholism, temptations, addictions, bad habits, dysfunction, and the like)* or anything that takes our minds, thoughts, will, or emotions away from the true knowledge of Christ—and *WHO WE ARE IN CHRIST!* (See chapter 15, "Affirmations")—come out only by prayer and fasting.

In this book, that is what we will explore: *a commitment to getting well and a scientific formula for intermittent fasting + lots of water + lots of prayer—to learn how to develop meditation, patience, perseverance, self-control, and faithfulness as you go through The A.N.G.E.L. Plan©, **and to also realize that you already have the Holy Spirit that lives within You** if you have accepted Jesus Christ as your Savior, Lord and Master.*

As you get well, you will find that the various fruits of the Spirit[2] *also begin manifesting in your mind, your nature, your character, and begin changing bad habits.* **(Only God can change us; we cannot change ourselves!)**

The Holy Spirit changes us through the **daily study of God's Word and our surrender of our own stubborn wills to the will of God**, which the Holy Spirit teaches us after we are reborn in Christ.

---

[2] "[T]he fruit of the Spirit is love, joy, peace, patience, kindness, goodness, faithfulness, gentleness, self-control" (Galatians 5:22–23 NJKV).

COMMENT: You will find as you read **The A.N.G.E.L. Plan**© some repetition of certain scriptures or basic principles. ***REPETITION STRENGTHENS AND CONFIRMS HABIT, AND FAITH BECOMES NATURAL!*** *Not scriptural, but a definite truth!*

INTRODUCTION
How it All Began

One day he [the serpent] asked the woman, "Did God really say you must not eat the fruit from any of the trees in the garden?"

"Of course, we may eat fruit from the trees in the garden," said the woman. "It's only the fruit from the tree in the middle of the garden that we are not allowed to eat. God said, "You must not eat it or even touch it; if you do, you will die."

"You won't die!" the serpent replied to the woman. God knows that your eyes will be opened as soon as you eat it, and you will be like God, knowing both good and evil."

The woman was convinced. She saw that the tree was beautiful, and its fruit looked delicious, and **she wanted** the wisdom it would give her. **So, she took some of the fruit and ate it. Then she gave some to her husband, who was with her, and he ate it too.**

At that moment, their eyes were opened, and they suddenly felt **shame at their nakedness.**

So, they sewed fig leaves together to cover themselves. (Genesis 3:1–7 NLT)

Just imagine if we made a list of all times we have tried, or have actually covered, our shame and nakedness, physically and spiritually—how long would that list be?

Eve had a choice, and she chose to satisfy the desires of the flesh! Adam had a choice and followed his fleshly nature too!

Oh, how much we need Jesus!

1

The Lord's Priorities

(1) We should love the Lord our God with all our hearts, strength, mind, and spirit; and (2) we should love our neighbor as we love ourselves (Matthew 22:37, 39 NKJV). **That supersedes everything!**

Concerning how we are to conduct ourselves in our personal daily lives, our soul, our relationship with God, and with others, and how to stay healthy, Jesus taught the people in this order, according to Matthew 6, during His Sermon on the Mount:

1. How to **GIVE**,
2. How to **PRAY** and then He taught them The Lord's Prayer
3. How to **FORGIVE**
4. How to **FAST**

FASTING is right up there in the **top four things that Jesus told us to do and how to do it:**

Give. Pray. Forgive. Fast.
Give. Pray. Forgive. Fast.
Give. Pray. Forgive. Fast…

The Word of God teaches us that we are not to be boastful about our fasting, but to do it in secret before God.

In Matthew 6:16–18, Jesus commanded,

> And **when** you fast, don't make it obvious, as the hypocrites do, for they try to look miserable and disheveled so people will admire them for their fasting. I tell you the truth, that is the only reward they will ever get.
>
> But when you fast, comb your hair and wash your face.
>
> Then no one will notice that you are fasting, except your Father, who knows what you do in private. **And your Father, who sees everything, will reward you.** (NLT)

You will find such fasting easier and easier to do as you realize that it is GOD who is enabling you to fast through A New Godly Eating Lifestyle and by feasting on His Word. *Solicit the help of your household members to not tempt you when you're fasting.* If they don't always cooperate, forgive them immediately. Sometimes you just have to have a very firm "NO." Do it with love.

Don't get haughty or overly religious about it whatever you do. They will learn from you that *The A.N.G.E.L. Plan*© brings many more changes than healing the thyroid and weight loss!

May the **Holy Spirit of Jesus Christ** flood you with patience for yourself and give you an anointing to understand, accept, commit to, and fully embrace *The A.N.G.E.L. Plan*©!

You definitely will not be disappointed!

2

Our Despair

Have you ever just wanted to die?

Have you known what it is to wake up to the feeling of shame, annoyance, physical or emotional pain, utter humiliation? All because of what you stuffed in your mouth yesterday?

Firmly resolving to do better today and then tomorrow, to start over, to extremely diet, to exercise…on and on and on….

To go all day without a morsel in your mouth—to make up for what you ate yesterday?

To purge?

To totally fast?

To colon cleanse, total cleanse, diet pills, fat blockers, fat burners, carb blockers?

To eat only protein, fat-free, carb-free, egg whites, dry salads, veggies only?

Keto diet, paleo, Daniel's plan, Atkins, Scarsdale, South Beach Diet, the Zone? Too many to count or keep up with!

Diuretics, starvation, liquids only, protein bars only, vegan only, whey, protein shakes, or smoothies only?

Join the gym, jazzercise, aerobics, planking, martial arts, Pilates, or exercise three times daily to perhaps lose ten pounds before a life event?

Take up CrossFit, running, jogging, walking, hiking…limping?

Health spas, fat farms, rehab programs, therapists, twelve-step programs?

As a Christian, have you ever tried to **pray or bless the calories away** in whatever you're about to consume? *I have plenty of times.*

Do you secretly think that you're unique, that God will allow you to eat unhealthy and fattening things and it won't add to fat on your body? That you're the one person who will get by with it?

Or have you been tempted to just give up? To go on eating like you had been—or even worse?

MAKE NO MISTAKE: WE REAP WHAT WE SOW!

If we sow unhealthy foods into our body, we will reap fat and poor health!

How do I know? I've thought the same things, held the same attitudes, felt the same insane feelings. I also believed that I was a special case, unique—unfortunately "terminally unique" as we say in recovery.

My soul and body were slowly dying from all of my own attempts and seemingly hard work to lose weight…and what anguish…**what anguish!**

3

Gluttony

(What the Bible Says)

Do you like honey?
Don't eat too much,
or it will make you sick!"
It's not good to eat too much honey,
and it's not good to
seek honors for yourself.
A person without self-control is
like a city with broken-down walls.
(Proverbs 25:16, 27–28 NLT)

What does that mean to you—"a city with broken-down walls?" To me, it means total **lack of self-discipline and no physical defense** against any attacks of satan!

The fruit of self-control is one that we already have within us! At our new birth in Christ, we are given the seeds of all of the fruit of the Spirit to be developed in God's timing. This means that we already have spirits of power, love, and self-control (a sound mind), which is our first and best defense!

How sad that we might be overcome by the temptations of the flesh when Jesus returns, or on any day that we allow ourselves to be overcome by the worries and desires of the flesh and ignore the presence of His Holy Spirit within us.

Jesus is our daily bread and our Living Water!

How can we so easily forget?

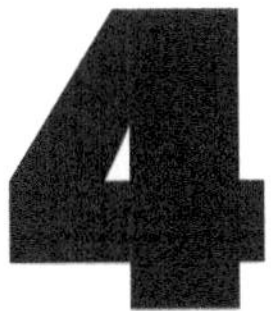

More on Fasting

Before you begin fasting, Jesus said,

> **Put oil on your head and
> wash your face so that your
> fasting will not be noticed by people,
> but by your Father who is in secret;
> and your Father who sees in secret
> will reward you.**
> (Matthew 6:17–18 AMP)

You will find fasting in secret easier and easier to do as you realize that it is **GOD who is enabling you to adapt** to *A New Godly Eating Lifestyle©*, and we are changed by feasting on His Word.

With that in mind, **when you begin** *The A.N.G.E.L. Plan©*, you may find it wise to **discuss with your housemates your intention to adapt to** *The A.N.G.E.L. Plan©*. Take time to explain to them what you are doing and **ask them specifically to NOT tempt you to eat when you're fasting**.

If they do tempt you without thinking or consciously doing so, don't hold it against them or ever get mad at them. Just reiterate your choice of *The A.N.G.E.L. Plan©*. Our close people often don't know how to react to *A New Godly Eating Lifestyle©*.

Of course, you may be flexible some days, but other days, your housemates need to really understand your firm "no" or "not now."

As they see your results of *The A.N.G.E.L. Plan©*, they may want to join you too!

The point of this scripture, I think, is to tell us that **we are not to announce to the world that we are fasting by looking morose or dejected or "put upon," but instead, we should rejoice in the Lord!**

This is OUR CHOICE OF EATING LIFESTYLE!

Jesus told us to fast in Matthew 6 during His Sermon on the Mount. He taught the people in this order, to GIVE, PRAY, FORGIVE, FAST.

Fasting is as important to God as praying, giving, and forgiving!

5

Eating Disorderly Hell

Compulsive Overeating and **The Diet Rollercoaster**

My first diet started when I was ten years old, when I put on my red polka-dot bathing suit, and my uncle told me I needed to go on a diet. **Shame, self-hatred, me, myself, and I ALL** got on the diet rollercoaster that day for the first time.

When I was sixteen, my father started taking diet pills, and I asked if I could take them too. Mama said no, but Daddy said yes (that's the way I operated—play them against each other or go with the answer that I wanted to hear). I then started taking my first "diet pills"—little yellow capsules—and I loved the way it felt. For at least twenty-five years, I battled with many kinds of prescription diet pills and every over-the-counter vitamin or weight loss supplement or over-the-counter drug as they became available.

As far as I was concerned, I had tried everything and listened to everybody to find a way out of my battle with food.

Of course, my own battle with food became more urgent, and it just got worse and worse. *I was successful at times, but more times than not, I failed miserably!*

Here are some of the things I learned about all eating disorders that I'd like to share with you.

Bulimia Nervosa

We look to the Mayo Clinic for the definition:

> Bulimia nervosa, commonly called bulimia, is a serious, potentially life-threatening eating disorder. People with bulimia may secretly binge—eating large amounts of food with a loss of control over the eating—and then purge, trying to get rid of the extra calories in an unhealthy way. (https://www.mayoclinic.org/diseases-conditions)

In the early nineties, I had a couple of years of mild bulimia where I would either eat everything on one day and fast completely the next, or where I would eat until I was sick, purge, and start eating again…repeatedly… I even took serums to help myself upchuck. I want to thank GOD for thirty-four years in twelve-step programs, including a year in Overeaters Anonymous, for helping me out of the dung pit of bulimia!

My heart goes out to those who have previously, or are currently dealing with, bulimia, as I have seen bulimia a lot worse than I ever had it.

Without knowing she had bulimia, I rented a room in my house to an acquaintance I'll call Stella. Only two nights passed before I discovered Stella's bulimia in all of its ugly stages. In her room were food bags everywhere, new food in one corner, trash in another corner. I remember Stella eating all the food she could eat and then upchuck and start all over again all throughout the night. It was impossible to sleep through it since we had adjacent rooms and a common bathroom.

My friend was anemic, thin, and all the stomach bile and acid had made her beautiful, perfect teeth translucent—you could actually see through them!

God meant that I live with her during her extreme sickness so that I would abruptly say to myself and to God, "NOOOOO! Lord, I don't ever want to go there!"

When I saw Stella again about a year later, she had finally recovered through the twelve-step programs. Stella looked healthy and beautiful and told me she was going to get her teeth fixed! Praise God! Thank you, Jesus, our deliverer!

Anorexia Nervosa

Research tells me that the **(1) failure to eat enough food and (2) being overconscious of the physical appearance are the first signs of anorexia.**

> According to the website of the Mayo Clinic, "The physical signs and symptoms of Anorexia Nervosa are related to starvation. Anorexia also includes emotional and behavioral issues involving an **unrealistic perception of body weight** and **an extremely strong fear of gaining weight or becoming fat."** (https://www.mayoclinic.org/diseases-conditions)

Anorexia is a subject that I personally know little about other than pictures I've seen and people that I've seen that look impossibly thin, like they're sick or dying. Many of us remember our beloved Karen Carpenter, who, though rich and famous, was so anorexic it became fatal. Fatal to Karen and fatal to The Carpenters.

Body Dysmorphic Disorder

Body dysmorphic disorder is something I'm familiar with from my personal experiences—a flaw that appears minor or really can't be seen by others. Mayo Clinic defines body dysmorphic disorder as,

> Body dysmorphic disorder is a mental health condition in which one can't stop thinking about one or more perceived defects or flaws in their appearance—a flaw that appears minor or can't

be seen by others." (https://www.mayoclinic.org/ diseases-conditions)

Having battled food on the diet rollercoaster for over forty years, I know the pain, disappointment, and disgust that make us hate ourselves, **as well as the deceptions and deceit that satan causes when we look in the mirror.**

One brief look in the mirror may either start our day off well or may send us into a downward spiral that may not be easy to stop!

I know from experience that when one does lose weight, body dysmorphic disorder may tell us either that we haven't lost a thing, or—wow!—that we lost thirty pounds yesterday!

We can either become the wallflower of the day, or we try to stuff ourselves into clothes three sizes too small in order to get attention and flattery.

A celebrated singer, dancer, and musician was so overcome by body dysmorphic disorder that he changed his face many times yet couldn't face his own disorders.

Body dysmorphic disorder only truly gets better if you can give it to God and ask Him to keep your perception true and accurate. And bind the devil from your perceptions, your mind, and your mirror!

6

My Freedom Story

So much to tell, yet I'll stick to my battle with food and its control over me. Over forty years of struggling with food, various diets, food choices, overeating, binging, completely fasting…with some success—but it was usually a yo-yo thing!

Up and down the scales I'd go within a one-hundred-pound range! So please allow me to touch on the parts of my story that brought me to freedom from my food obsession.

I was born in southwest Louisiana in the wake of Hurricane Audrey. My father had dubbed me "*the little mistake*" before I was ever born (because my siblings were eighteen and thirteen when I came along). I wasn't planned nor wanted by my father. That misnomer and nickname "the little mistake" stayed with me for at least my first three years.

Even after my father had stopped calling me *the little mistake*, those words rang through my brain many times as a child, as a teenager, and on into adulthood. It seemed I was set to prove that I was NO mistake, little or big. Often, I was obnoxious in doing so, and for that I apologize to all whom I've hurt with my old behavior.

Like so many of us, my parents were dysfunctional, but they were nonetheless good parents to me—but that's *their* story and will not be my excuse for eating, overeating, and stuffing my feelings any more. Suffice it to say, **I grew up learning that home-cooked food and ice cream could soothe the strife and tension in our house.**

My parents, to whom I was born late in life (forty-four and thirty-seven), pretty much despised each other yet remained married and together for forty-eight years.

There was constant arguing and cursing, and my mother had no trust in my father and for good reason. I prayed they'd get a divorce so they would stop arguing. When I was a small child, I remember hiding in the closet when they started arguing and particularly when my father came in at 2:00 or 3:00 a.m. It seemed to my toddler mind that all hell broke loose! My dad would end the argument by ignoring Mama or just going to bed, and she would go on accepting his behavior year after year…

I swore to myself that I would never let my children live like that.

My first diet started at the age of ten. My uncle told me that I needed to go on a diet, and I began to feel shame and self-hatred. I got on the diet rollercoaster for the first time that day.

When I was at the ripe old age of sixteen, my father started taking diet pills, and I asked if I could take them too. I did, and I loved the way it felt. I then began the battle with prescription and over-the-counter diet pills on and off for the next twenty-five years.

Then came a couple of years of mild bulimia, from which I was delivered by God and through Overeaters Anonymous in 1992.

My battle with food became more urgent, and I was successful at times, but more times than not, I failed miserably.

After yo-yo dieting for over forty years, I begged God to help one more time… It felt like something had changed in me spiritually, and God heard my prayer!

My story continues in various places in this book, as I explain what works for me and others.

7

Compiling

THE A.N.G.E.L. PLAN
A New Godly Eating Lifestyle©

After yo-yo dieting on and off for over forty years, in January of 2018, I again begged God to help me.

BUT THIS TIME, I felt like something had changed in me spiritually and God heard my prayer! As I began to THANK HIM for a rejuvenated faith, I envisioned myself with a thin, rejuvenated body!

I continued to visualize my new image every time I looked in a mirror or when I was discouraged. I learned to THANK GOD for the answers to my prayers and visualized them coming into fruition (fruits of the Spirit). That made all the difference!

Step back a bit. For the previous four years beginning in 2014, I had begun researching and recording every scripture that I could find that pertained to food, gluttony, God's strength and hope, and His New Testament commandments about eating, drinking, fasting, and feasting. I accumulated fifty-seven single-spaced pages of scripture and a few commentaries, and I recorded all the scriptures and listened to them over and over, yet the battle with food and the dance with diets continued.

It just wasn't coming together for me. *I was missing something—* some component that would allow success and victory over the hellish battle with food.

The next few years slowly passed, and major depression (especially at the death of my sister) came and went in various stages.

I would wake up every day to start beating myself up over what I ate the day before, yet looking forward to that day's food and that night's bowl of ice cream.

Toward the end, I would buy out Safeway's frozen yogurt (in an ice cream carton) and binge on it at night. I would buy four half-gallons of them at a time—and then worry that I would run out! The most I weighed before *The A.N.G.E.L. Plan*© was up to 245 pounds!

My solution was to throw away the scales! (This has served me well throughout *The A.N.G.E.L. Plan*© too).

If you can get away from the scales as evidence of your progress and go with what you actually feel (newly found muscles or bones, like ribs, hipbones, backbones, etc.), **how your clothes slowly begin to get looser and looser on you—and ultimately your new smaller clothes, let that be your measure of progress—not some silly, usually off scales that don't ever agree with any doctor's scales!**

Having read and tried everything I could think of to get rid of the pounds, one day I ran across a woman's magazine (the name of which I cannot remember) with an article discussing scientific research revealing that **intermittent fasting (7 hours eating and 17 fasting) could start healing one's thyroid in two days!** Wow—I had been using two different types of thyroid medication for over twenty-five years! **I had to try it!**

The article also said that if I did **intermittent fasting four to five days a week that I would begin to lose weight. Really?** Nothing else had worked!

I tried intermittent fasting for a week or so and saw no results—again!

I could not stick to it by myself. I needed some help—something more.

A couple of weeks later, during my prayer time, the Lord impressed on me to do the following:

1) Take the **7/17-hour intermittent fasting process** described earlier.
2) Combine it with four to six 16-oz **glasses or bottles of water daily**.
3) **At the same time, add the most important ingredients**:

   a. **Prayer with supplication** (specific requests) and
   b. *Thanksgiving for what God has ALREADY done and IS doing,* **and devotions and meditation throughout the day, in both times of fasting and times for eating.**

Fast for the things that God puts on your heart each day, or simply for health or weight loss and riddance of our body dysmorphic disorders.

Out of desperation and a newfound sense of hope that I might one day win the battle of FOOD SLAVERY, I began to **hope** this three-prong approach might actually free my mind of thinking about food all the time—all past, present, and future eating.

I *knew* how to eat right and what to eat—I knew all the "right" diet foods, but alone, I just could not do it. Yet now I began to have **hope**!

I prayed and asked God to anoint me in what has become *The A.N.G.E.L. Plan*©. And I began with a fervor, if for no other reason than to heal my thyroid!

In the next four months, with extraordinarily little exercise other than walking my dogs the shortest distance possible, **God removed forty pounds!**

After the first three months, I began to feel light-headed and went to my internist. **The doctor told me that we needed to remove** one of my two thyroid medications that I had been on for twenty-five years because my thyroid was beginning to function again!

After six months, I began to feel light-headed again and removed the second twenty-five-year thyroid medication! **My thyroid was truly healed.**

WOW! IT WORKED: THE A.N.G.E.L. PLAN FULLY HEALED MY THYROID!

The three-prong approach, The A.N.G.E.L. Plan©, *actually worked!* 7/17 FASTING + LOTS OF WATER + LOTS OF DAILY PRAYER WITH SUPPLICATION AND IMMEDIATE THANKSGIVING, AND DEVOTIONS! So very simple!

The A.N.G.E.L. Plan© works!

I was completely off all thyroid medication for the first time in twenty-five years, and in every thyroid test since then, my thyroid hormone results are all in normal ranges!

By the end of the first year, God removed over eighty pounds and ten pants sizes! ALL PRAISE BE TO GOD!

*By the grace and mercy of God, I now do this each week, and it truly is a new eating lifestyle for me—**not some quick weight loss, yo-yo diet** that I can "fall off of" or break or screw up, etc.!*[3]

I'll explain more in the "Devotions" section of this book about how to go about *The A.N.G.E.L. Plan©* successfully. **It is really important that you begin reading chapter 12, the "Devotions" section, right away.** I even suggest that you read all the devotions

---

[3] There was a time when I stopped *The A.N.G.E.L. Plan©* completely (my husband said I was "too thin"), and I soon regretted it. It took me a while and pounds found until I could completely resubmit myself to the daily anointing of *The A.N.G.E.L. Plan©*! Now that I've been fully back for two years now, I pray God I will *never* ever give up on *The A.N.G.E.L. Plan: A New Godly Eating Lifestyle©*! And those found pounds are gone. Praise God!

early on so you more fully understand the beauty of *The A.N.G.E.L. Plan©*! Then focus on one devotion at a time.

My intercession for you will continue, even though I may not know you. I pray that God will anoint you and give you the sense of urgency, opportunity, and His timing to start *The A.N.G.E.L. Plan©*!

May you be truly blessed and have miraculous results!

SOME OF THE MANY BENEFITS OF
INTERMITTENT FASTING

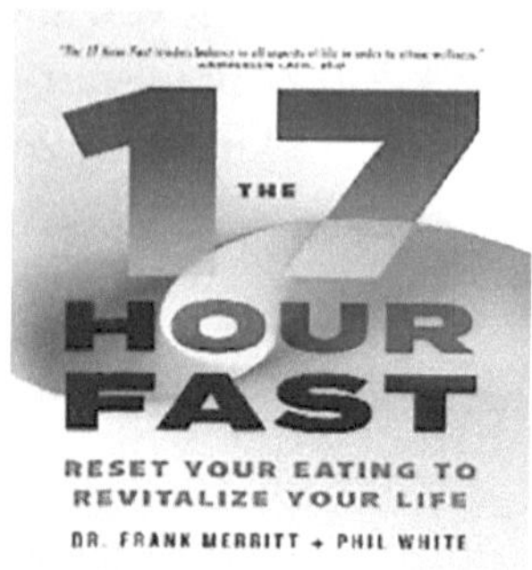

The following is what I have gleaned from reading and studying various Bible verses, articles on intermittent fasting, the importance of enough daily water intake, and my own experience. The first I read was the woman's magazine mentioned earlier that discussed the fact that a 7/17 fast, if done for as few as TWO DAYS, will begin to heal your thyroid.

Secondly, I read in *The 17 Hour Fast: Reset Your Eating to Revitalize Your Life* by Dr. Frank Merritt and Phil White (May 13, 2018) that the 7/17 fast can help anyone:

- Cut cholesterol, reduce bacterial overgrowth, and lower toxins;
- Start making lifestyle changes that lower body weight and BMI and reduce body fat;
- Improve digestive issues like IBS, fatty liver disease, and acid reflux;
- Boost physical and cognitive performance;
- Break free from habitual and boredom-related eating;
- Create a rich, fully-engaged experience before, during, and after fasting;
- Achieve many of the benefits of a 48-hour fast in less than half that time, while avoiding many of the pitfalls and risks of more extreme fasts;

- Overcome food-related psychological and behavioral issues while turning destructive habits into healthy ones;
- Reduce sugar dependence;
- Achieve more restful and restorative sleep; and
- Use fasting to strengthen work-life balance and improve one's relationships.

This is all *in addition to* healing the thyroid and a healthy weight loss!

8

Why Do We Need Devotions?

Do not be conformed to this world,
but be transformed by the
renewing of your mind,
that you may prove what is that good and
acceptable and perfect will of God.
(Romans 12:2 NKJV)

God said that we are to be transformed by the renewing of our mind through His Word. That transformation is something only God can truly do as we learn more of His word and of how it speaks to those struggling with eating disorders and other addictions.

Devotions remind us to spend time daily in prayer and in the Word and to focus on *The A.N.G.E.L. Plan©* *before* we start eating for that day. When we do, it's so much easier to embrace and commit to *A New Godly Eating Lifestyle©*.

I highly recommend that you read through all the devotions at once and you will learn much more about *The A.N.G.E.L. Plan©*.

9

A Few of God's Promises

NO TEMPTATION IS GREATER THAN YOU IN CHRIST!

*No temptation has overtaken you
except such as is common to mankind.
And God is faithful; He will not let you be
tempted beyond what you can bear!*
**But when you are tempted,
*HE WILL ALSO PROVIDE
A WAY OUT
SO THAT YOU CAN ENDURE IT.***
(1 Corinthians 10:13 NIV)

**GOD GIVES AND
RENEWS OUR STRENGTH**

***I can do all things through
Christ Who strengthens me!***
(Philippians 4:13 NKJV)

Just think of all the possibilities! If God has a task for us, Christ will give us strength to accomplish it to its end. *Selah.*

"Don't be afraid, for I am with you.
Don't be discouraged, for I am your God.

I will strengthen you and help you.
I will hold you up with
My Victorious Right Hand."
*"For **I hold you by your right hand—***
I, the Lord your God.
*And I say to you, **"'Don't be afraid.***
I AM here to HELP YOU.'"
(Isaiah 41:10,13 NLT)

Have you not known? Have you not heard?
The Lord is the everlasting God,
the Creator of the ends of the earth.
He does not faint or grow weary;
His understanding is unsearchable.
He gives power to the faint,
and to him who has no might
He increases strength.
(Isaiah 40:28–41 NIV)

BUT THOSE WHO WAIT ON THE LORD
SHALL RENEW THEIR STRENGTH;
they shall mount up with wings like eagles;
they shall run and not be weary;
they shall walk and not faint.
(Isaiah 40:31 NKJV)

In Matthew 7:7–8 (NLT), Jesus said,

Keep on asking, *and*
you will receive what you ask for.
Keep on seeking, *and you will find.*
Keep on knocking,
and the door will be opened to you.
For everyone who asks, receives.
Everyone who seeks, finds.
And to everyone who knocks,
the door will be opened.

NO MORE HUNGER OR THIRST

"I will say to the prisoners,
'Come out in freedom,'
and to those in darkness,
'Come into the light.'
They will be My sheep,
grazing in green pastures
and on hills that were previously bare.
They will neither hunger nor thirst...."
(Isaiah 49:9–10 NLT)

In John 6:35 (AMPC), Jesus promised,

I am the Bread of Life.
He who comes to Me
will never be hungry,
and he who believes in and
cleaves to and trusts in and relies
on Me will never thirst anymore.

In Matthew 6:16–18 (NLT), Jesus instructed,

And when you fast, don't make it obvious,
as the hypocrites do, for they try to look miser-
able and disheveled so people will admire them
for their fasting. I tell you the truth, that is the
only reward they will ever get.

But when you fast, comb your hair and
wash your face.

Then no one will notice that you are fast-
ing, except your Father, who knows what you
do in private. And your Father, who sees every-
thing, will reward you.

10

Fat is a Family Affair

If you were raised by parents who tended to be overweight and your siblings are also fluffy, you may have seen food addiction in your immediate household. Perhaps you accepted overeating and being fluffy as just the way things were, and no one made you the wiser.

That doesn't have to be true anymore! You can leave your old lifestyle of food addiction and the dance with diets in the dust!

God led me into compiling this manuscript for *The A.N.G.E.L. Plan: A New Godly Eating Lifestyle*© to set us free from slavery to food, which will eventually lead us naturally into really healthy food choices.

In my lifetime, I have tried all the many different diets—fad diets and crash diets…*ad nauseum.* No matter what I had seriously tried, it seems at least one member of my immediate household has tried to sabotage my dieting or fasting efforts in some little—or big—way.

You can also expect the same from one or more of your household members or colleagues or schoolmates even now, even though you are committed to *The A.N.G.E.L. Plan*©.

When, for their own reasons, someone either consciously or subconsciously sabotages your daily commitment to *The A.N.G.E.L. Plan*©, stop, pray, and get direction and strength from God to stick to your commitment that day. There is no need to call their attention to their sabotage, just make a firm "NO," whether it be verbally or mentally. One of my husband's favorite things to do is cook bacon often in the morning, which is during my fasting period! Wow, does that take God's strength!

Remember that God never tempts us, but **we are led astray by our own selfish desires.** James 1:13–14 (NIV) says,

> *When tempted, no one should say,*
> *"God is tempting me."*
> *For God cannot be tempted by evil,*
> *nor does He tempt anyone;*
> *but each person is tempted*
> *when they are dragged away by*
> *their own evil desire and enticed.*

If you have committed to fast but then don't, or you have an unscheduled "eating event" that is not part of your daily commitment, then you have NOT FAILED. YOU CANNOT FAIL! You just haven't fasted that day. This is *A New Godly Eating Lifestyle*©, not some yo-yo diet! You can simply fast the next day if you want!

11

"The A.N.G.E.L. Plan©"

Of course, *The A.N.G.E.L. Plan©* begins with prayer! Jesus began in Matthew 6:9–13 (NKJV),

> *In this manner, therefore, pray:*
> *"Our Father in heaven,*
> *hallowed be Your name.*
> *Your kingdom come.*
> *Your will be done on earth*
> *as it is in Heaven.*
> *Give us this day our daily bread.*
> *And forgive us our debts,*
> *as we forgive our debtors.*
> *And do not lead us into temptation*
> *but deliver us from the evil one.*
> *For Yours is the kingdom and the power*
> *and the glory, now and forever!*
> *Amen.*

Remember, *The A.N.G.E.L. Plan©* is SIMPLE!

1. **Commit your day to God and** *A New Godly Eating Lifestyle.* **Thank Him that you no longer have to be on any diet or looking for the latest fad in dieting! Just stop for a moment to feel the freedom of not having to diet**

ever again! You literally ***give up dieting*** because YOU have a new eating *LIFESTYLE!* **Ask for God's anointing early in the day!**

2. **Eat sensibly for 7 hours a day and fast the other 17 hours. During your fasting periods, you may drink water, coffees, teas, or zero-calorie drinks—as long as they have no nutritional value. REMEMBER, IT'S NOT *WHAT* YOU EAT SO MUCH AS IT IS *WHEN* YOU EAT!**

3. **Determine how many days you want to fast each week. According to my early research and my *own experience*, two days in a row should heal your thyroid and restart your metabolism *(see chapter 6, "MY FREEDOM STORY")*.**

   If you're interested in weight loss, choose to fast three to five days a week. This is not a hard and "fast" rule (excuse the pun). **It's best that you do "set your mind" to a predetermined number of days of the week. Select what days you feel led or want to fast and what daily times work best for your schedule.**

   This may change daily depending on your scheduling needs, **yet always listen for God before you start eating for the day! And remember, fasting includes sleeping time!**

4. **Drink six sixteen-ounce of bottles of water a day. It may take you time to build up to this but keep trying. It becomes a lot easier in just two or three days. Add lemon or zest! *WATER IS ABSOLUTELY ESSENTIAL to The A.N.G.E.L. Plan© and cannot be overemphasized! Water, water, and more water to, among many other things, flush the toxins out and to help rid your body of its burned fat through ketosis.***

5. **Pick one feast day of the week** (I pick Sunday) **and stick with that. Let that be the day on which you don't fast but will enjoy everything you eat that day, guilt-free and in the fruit of the spirit of self-control.** I also consider holidays as feast days.

6. **Don't be foolish! If you're fasting three to five days a week to promote weight loss, certainly you can enjoy**

and eat what you'd like during your feast times, *but if you stuff yourself with unhealthy foods or snacks, you will seriously hamper your weight loss*—or even gain weight! PRAY FOR WISDOM IN EATING DURING YOUR FEASTING PERIODS!

7. REMEMBER: If you have committed to fast but then don't, or you have a special "eating event" that is not part of your daily commitment, then you have NOT FAILED. You just haven't fasted that day. This is *A New Godly Eating Lifestyle©,* not some yo-yo diet! You can simply fast the next day! YOU CANNOT FAIL UNLESS YOU STOP TRYING! FAILURE IS NOT NECESSARY!

BONUS: If you want to really speed up your weight loss and increase your body strength, add the dreaded "E" word to your vocabulary and daily life. Exercise always helps but *exercise is not mandatory!* Just start moving around at first, asking Christ to let you step into His yoke, you take the first step, and the next steps become much easier as He takes over...and the next step and the next and the next....

Go for the gusto and SET YOUR MIND! As you slim down, you'll be encouraged and will definitely want to start moving. You will be absolutely AMAZED at how easy exercise can be WHEN YOU TAKE THE FIRST STEP AND LET JESUS TAKE THE NEXT!

Prayer

Thank you, Father, for The A.N.G.E.L. Plan: A New Godly Eating Lifestyle©! *Help me, Lord, as only You and Your Word can do!*
I ask that You anoint me to do The A.N.G.E.L. Plan© *for healing of my body and for weight loss, and I ask that You make it a permanent new lifestyle for me—and I* thank You *that* my Prayer is already answered!*—and its manifestation is already happening! In the name of Jesus, amen!*

12

Devotions

1

From the ends of the earth,
I cry to You for help
when my heart is overwhelmed.
Lead me to the towering rock of safety,
for You are my safe refuge,
a fortress where my enemies
cannot reach me.
(Psalm 61:2–3 NLT)

How often have we begged God—both in the secret places of our heart and out loud—or really loud—to deliver us from the bondage of food addiction? I have more than a thousand times over my lifetime.

But then, after four years of biblical research on what God thinks about eating and the place of food in our lives, God showed me *The A.N.G.E.L. Plan*, based on the Word of God and scientific research. *(See chapter 6, "My Freedom Story.")*

The A.N.G.E.L. Plan© is not for everyone. **It works for anyone who has absolutely reached the end of their rope after trying all known methods to defeat the battle with "food as fuel" versus "food as pleasure" and satisfaction of our emotions.**

If you live your life devoted to God and are willing to lean on Him and His Word in good times as well as the tough times, then *The A.N.G.E.L. Plan©* will work for you!

Prayer: Father God, in the name of Jesus, hear my prayer and help me to submit to Your Word in everything that I think, do, say, imagine, plan, speak, or express.
I pray and fast today for:

____

____

____

*I know that I am not alone in this battle, but that **You and I can defeat this enemy with the Word of God and the fruit of the Holy Spirit.** Amen and amen.*

2

Don't people complain about unsalted food?
Does anyone want the tasteless white of an egg?
My appetite disappears when I look at it;
I gag at the thought of eating it!
(Job 6:6–7 NLT)

None of us who have battled with food actually enjoy being on a special diet or having to eat "low cal" and "low fat" or "no fat" or "low carb" or diet, bland, tasteless foods. It is restrictive and unsatisfying and not any kind of a long-term solution to the problems of overeating, obesity, and fat.

That's not how God designed you to live at all! Christ died to set us free from the law of sin and death and to break the power of the enemy over us, the constant "thorn in the side." He does not want us to live in a constant mental, physical, emotional, and spiritual battle against fat, obesity, breathing, and walking problems, along with physical and emotional sicknesses that come from constantly being bombarded by or enslaved to thoughts of food.

We fail to see, or cannot see yet, that food is given to us to be used as fuel and for our health and enjoyment—but NOT to suppress or relieve our constant needs for relief of boredom, loneliness, low self-esteem, guilt, shame, and general dissatisfaction with life. Food is fuel. That's it.

Prayer: Father, in the holy, mighty, and powerful name of Jesus, I ask You—and I thank You already—for opening this new door to A New Godly Eating Lifestyle: The A.N.G.E.L. PLAN© I thank You that I can find peace and freedom from food addiction by following this simple and easy new eating lifestyle.

I pray and fast today for:

____

____

____

I thank You that already You have anointed me to move into A New Godly Eating Lifestyle© *that blesses and glorifies You and that heals me, body, mind, thoughts, soul, and spirit. Amen.*

3

So, let's not get tired of doing what is good.
At just the right time we will reap
a harvest of blessing if we don't give up.
(Galatians 6:9 NLT)

About the thi[rd] or four[th] day of the A.N.G.E.L. plan, perhaps you feel like you just couldn't fast that day.
You have two choices, both of which are excellent:

- You can turn to God as humbly as you know how today and seek His face until you know what path will bring peace in your "gut" that day—not only peace in your heart, but peace to your physical body. **Overeating does not bring peace—because gluttony is a sin**. Sometimes you will have to seek Him minute by minute, whereas other times you instinctively know whether you are to fast or not that particular day.

  OR

- You can choose not to fast at all that day, and it's perfectly okay if you have peace in your gut about it. This is also where you can make room for special dinner plans, appointments, holidays, or vacation days.

YOU have choices. Choose PEACE. Every time.

Prayer: Father in the most holy name of Jesus, help me today to choose either fasting or feasting according to Your will today. You know what will best benefit me, and You know what events are ahead today.

I pray and fast today for:

____

____

____

Help me to recognize and follow Your perfect peace. In the name of Jesus, amen.

4

Don't be afraid, for I am with you.
Don't be discouraged, for I am your God.
I will strengthen you and help you.
I will hold you up with
My Victorious Right Hand…
For I hold you by your right hand—
I, the Lord your God.
And I say "Don't be afraid.
I am here to help you."
(Isaiah 41:10, 13 NLT)

God did not say anywhere in His Word that people should count calories or fats or proteins or carbohydrates or grams or ounces. **God did not say that we are to completely abstain from food for any particular length of time**, other than when the prophets, kings or priests called for fasts in the Old Testament.

God did not tell us to wear a certain pants size or dress size or to try to live up to other people's standards when it comes to what we wear on the outside. *It is what flows from our insides that counts!* **Are you flowing God or are you flowing self-recrimination or pride?**

What God DID say is that we are to **fast and to pray, and Jesus specifically told us that some demons** (addictions, bad habits, diseases, dysfunction) anything that takes our minds from the knowledge of Christ—and who we are in Christ—**come out only by prayer and fasting. In doing so, we find our healing.**

And God tells us NOT to be afraid because He is with us, not to be discouraged because He is our God! He says He will strengthen us and help us, and that He will hold us up with HIS victorious right hand—JESUS!

And three verses later, the Word repeats the same reassurance that **we are not to fear because He is here to help us…each moment, each second, each minute of each hour of each day of**

each week of each month of each year of each decade—forever and ever. Amen!

*Prayer: Holy Father, in the mighty and glorious name of Jesus, **I give all of my fears and all my worries to You. Please handle them because I cannot. You see solutions where I see roadblocks. You have a plan to get around the roadblocks ahead in our lives.***
You know Your miracles, and I know You!
I pray and fast today for:

____

____

____

*Please help me as I learn to **eat to live instead of live to eat.** Open my eyes to the truths in The A.N.G.E.L. Plan©. In the mighty name of Jesus! Amen and amen.*

5

[T]hey who wait for the Lord
shall renew their strength;
they shall mount up with wings like eagles;
they shall run and not be weary;
they shall walk and not faint.
(Isaiah 40:31 ESV)

As I write this meditation today, we are in the beginning of the coronavirus pandemic. Fear threatens every move, and my newlywed husband is in California while I am in Arkansas. I feel very alone in a new city with but three of my dearest loved ones, my bonus daughter Alana and my best friends, Becky and Janet—yet not my newlywed husband, my son, nor my grandsons who are all back in California.

While food used to be my comforter, the Holy Ghost has now taken over that role, and I am NO LONGER ENSLAVED to my mental and physical appetites that would like to torture me.

Jesus said some "demons" come out only through prayer and fasting. Embracing intermittent fasting keeps you praying and puts you in a position to be rid of the enslavement to your appetites where, like me, you probably have been most of your life!

BUT if I wait on the Lord to intervene and renew my strength, my hope, my faith, my self-control, and self-discipline, I will also have the power of a **SOUND MIND!**

Prayer: **Holy Father, Lord Jesus, Holy Ghost, help me to pray today. Allow me to lean into You and lay at Your feet this burden I've been carrying for so long.**

Show me truths about myself that have kept me from **RUNNING TO YOU instead of running to food.** *Again. And again and again and again. And again.*

I pray and fast today for:

____

____

____

Keep me in the safe refuge of Your mighty fortress, oh, God, in the majestic and mighty name of Jesus, our Lord, our Savior, our healer, our master, our teacher and our king! Amen.

6

My son, as you go through life,
keep your appetite under control,
and **don't eat anything that**
you know is bad for you...
Don't feel that you just have to have
all sorts of fancy food, and
don't be a glutton over any food...
Gluttony has been the death of many people.
Avoid it and you'll live longer.
(Ecclesiastica)

It appears that for thousands and thousands of years, people have battled with food, "fancy foods" and gluttony. Gluttony not necessarily over all foods, but gluttony over any food.

For me, that would have been boiled crawfish, huge bowls of ice cream, ginger snaps, homemade butter-dripping popcorn, and chips and salsa. I still enjoy all of them, but I am no longer enslaved to any of them.

Jesus indicated that gluttony, among other kinds of sin *(through demons, unclean spirits, or addictions)*, **come out only by prayer and fasting.**

Enslavement to food, thoughts of food, plans of making food, or worrying about my next bite and where that will come from and when that will be... That enslavement, those thoughts, plans, and worries are long-gone from my psyche after following *The A.N.G.E.L. Plan*©—and eating the way God instructed us to eat.

Prayer: **Father, in the name of Jesus—the name that is above all names and to which every knee shall bow—***help me to enter into each time of prayer and fasting knowing that* **no temptation will come to me that You will not also provide a way out.**

I pray and fast today for:

____

____

____

Thank you for the blessings of freedom coming my way as I totally submit to **A New Godly Eating Lifestyle**©. *Amen and amen.*

7

*[K]eep on asking, and
you will receive what you ask for.
Keep on seeking,
and you will find.
Keep on knocking,
and the door will be opened to you.
For everyone who asks, receives.
Everyone who seeks, finds.
And to everyone who knocks,
the door will be opened.*
(Matthew 7:7–8 NLT)

Have you ever given up hope (whether you admit it to God or to yourself or not) that you will ever achieve self-discipline over food? I certainly have.

I read the Word and tried my hardest to believe the Word, and I knew that God had plans to give me hope and my future (Jeremiah 29:11), but I always kind of thought that the eating instructions in the Bible were for long ago.

Yet God's New Testament directions for fasting have not! The fasting instructions in God's Word are pertinent today, just as they were back then. **Jesus said, "When you fast…" not "IF you fast."**

God did not tell us in His Word to count calories, to have X number of grams of protein, nor to count carbohydrates and fats each day. He never mentioned those in His teachings on any eating lifestyle. He didn't suggest low carb, no sugar, low-fat or calculating proteins, micrograms, ounces, good or bad carbohydrates, ketones, ketosis, etc.

He did say that we are to pray and to fast, and that some things (evils) come out only by prayer and fasting.

Prayer: Father, in the name of Jesus, as I achieve my victory over enslavement to food, I ask that You never allow me to become haughty or proud of my physical results, but that I should always give You the glory for any positive changes in me. I cannot change myself, Lord—I've proven that over and over and over. It is only as I submit to You, using my sword of the Spirit of the Word, oh, God, and the principles of eating that You have set out in the Bible that I will come into the physical health that You desire for me to have.

I pray and fast today for:

____

____

____

As I pray and fast, may I realize that thousands of others are also praying and fasting at the same time, all for our good and Your glory! Amen!

8

Have you not known? Have you not heard?
The Lord is the everlasting God,
the Creator of the ends of the earth.
He does not faint or grow weary;
His understanding is unsearchable.
He gives power to the faint,
and to him who has no might, He increases strength.
Even youths shall faint and be weary,
and young men shall fall exhausted;
*but **they who wait for the Lord***
shall renew their strength;
they shall mount up with wings like eagles;
they shall run and not be weary;
they shall walk and not faint.
(Isaiah 40:28–41 ESV)

Amen! Bookmark this page! There is so much strength and encouragement from the Lord in this verse of God's Word. You have the power to resist temptation IF you believe that the Bible is true, and that God's Word provides strength to help YOU in ANY time of need or increased temptation.

God's *A.N.G.E.L. Plan* is different from other types of intermittent fasting because it incorporates God's Word and prayerful communication into our lives and our eating lifestyle—not only do we end up with a glorified body here in the present world (to be completely outshone when we reach heaven)—but **we restore HEALTH to our bodies and INCREASE OUR LONGEVITY here in the present world!**

Who doesn't want to be healthier, stronger, thinner, and more beautiful in this world? Certainly, YOU do!

Hang on, hang in there, hang tight, and **be still and know that the Lord is God...**

Prayer: Almighty Father, Jesus my Lord, my comforter and my strength, my indwelling Holy Ghost, please, please, please…JUST HELP ME!
I pray and fast today for:

____

____

____

I pray in the holy name of Jesus, amen and amen.

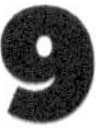

I will say to the prisoners,
"Come out in freedom,"
and to those in darkness,
"Come into the light."
They will be My sheep, grazing in green pastures
and on hills that were previously bare.
They will neither hunger nor thirst.
(Isaiah 49:9–10 NLT)

*YOU **CAN BE FREE** FROM SLAVERY TO FOOD!* **YES, YOU***!*

The A.N.G.E.L. Plan© quickly (within four to five days) becomes amazingly easy and then it becomes something that you WANT to do and CAN do for the rest of your life!

Isn't it wonderful to know that YOU, TOO, can enjoy the benefits of breaking that food addiction—that boredom addiction—that eternal craving to ingest food?

Often, we turn to food because we cannot control the situation around us, and excess food does absolutely NOTHING to help us improve spiritually, mentally, or physically. **There is nothing quite so physically intimate to us as ingesting food into our body—it becomes a part of us, and only you can make the decision to let God's Word work and to submit yourself to the guidance and leading of the Holy Spirit. He definitely WILL guide you and provide strength to help in your times of greatest temptation! JESUS is the Bread of Life and our Living Water!**

Prayer: My Dear Father, Jehovah Jirah! Abba, Father—my Daddy God, **thank you that You are more than willing to come immediately to my aid in times of temptation or hunger during my fasting periods,** *and please, Holy Spirit, keep me from overeating or thinking of junk food during my times of eating!*

Let my new **Godly eating lifestyle** *become second nature to me until it becomes my true nature!*

I love You and praise You and glorify You for who You are, my God, and I thank You that You alone are more than enough to give me the strength to do this today!

I pray and fast today for:

____

____

____

In the glorious name of Jesus, amen and amen!

10

[T]o keep me from becoming proud,
I was given a thorn in my flesh,
a messenger from satan to torment me and
keep me from becoming proud.
Three different times I begged the Lord to take it away.
Each time, He said, **"MY GRACE is all you need.**
MY POWER works best in weakness."
So now I am glad to boast about my weaknesses,
so that **the power of Christ can work through me.**
(2 Corinthians 12:7–9 NLT)

Like Paul, I had a thorn in my flesh that certainly kept me from becoming proud—the thorn of self-abuse, self-destruction, self-punishment, selfishness, selflessness, and certainly lacking the fruit of the spirit of self-control. **I lacked God's knowledge and wisdom when it came to my eating. I was unhappy with myself and others.**

We. Do. Every. Little. Thing. That. We. Can. Think. Of. to get those pounds off our body once and for all. We try until we have no more hope, no more willpower and little or no self-discipline or self-control, much less a sound mind when it comes to food!

Then we force ourselves into a position of utter hopelessness and are totally helpless to deal with our "thorn in the flesh" in our own strength.

What will I do in that place? **What will you do?**

Prayer: **Holy Father, in Jesus's mighty and precious name,** *I am utterly helpless in my own strength to deal with this thorn in my flesh of addiction to food and cravings that seem utterly overwhelming.* **May Your Holy Spirit lead me out of temptation and lead the way to my victory over food so that it no longer rules my thoughts, mind, will, or emotions; but that I see it as nothing other than fuel to my body.**

Jesus, You are the strength of my spirit, soul, and body! In Your strength, I can follow **The A.N.G.E.L. Plan!**
I pray and fast today for:

____

____

____

Amen and amen.

11

But HE said to me,
"MY grace is sufficient for you, for MY power is
made perfect in weakness."
Therefore, I will boast all the more gladly
about my weaknesses,
so that Christ's power may rest on me.
That is why, for Christ's sake,
I delight in weaknesses, in insults, in hardships,
in persecutions, in difficulties.
For when I am weak, then I am strong.
(2 Corinthians 12:9–10 NIV)

Jesus always, always, always encouraged people to look to Him for salvation, for mercy, for grace, for His strength through the Holy Ghost Who already dwells within us.

When we begin experiencing the physical manifestations of our A.N.G.E.L. plan in feeling and looking healthier or thinner, we can be so tempted to easily take credit for our successes ourselves when other people compliment us on how we look or act.

Be QUICK to put on His humility as you respond, **giving God the credit** for healing and changing your body's desires and eating habits.

The scriptures in this book are His Word, *The A.N.G.E.L. Plan*© is His idea that He planted in me over seven years ago!

*Prayer: Thank You, Father, that I am completely defeated when it comes to my own efforts at diets and diet programs—all to remove the fat evidence of gluttony from my body, which is Your temple. **For when I am weak, I run to YOU who is strong!***

Thank You, Father, that you have given me FREEDOM from the bondage of food and food addiction, and I will continue to heal and find strength in my body and my bones through hiding Your Word in my heart.

I give You my day, my mind, thoughts, will, emotions, words and expressions, actions and reactions—that I may be the person You want me to be for Your greatest glory.

I pray and fast today for:

____

____

____

In the name of Jesus! Amen.

12

Remember, when you are being tempted,
do not say, "God is tempting me."
God is never tempted to do wrong, and
He never tempts anyone else.
Temptation comes from our own desires
which entice us and drag us away.
(James 1:13–14 NLT)

But the Lord is faithful; and
HE will strengthen [setting you on a firm foundation] you and
protect and guard you from the evil one.
(2 Thessalonians 3:3 AMP)

When we're invited to a wedding, holiday party, a dinner party, a lunch date, a dinner date, or any kind of church or social or business gathering where food is an option, **we must know that our FIRST step should be to reach up and out to the Lord—breathe in God! Breathe in His strength and courage and remind yourself that God never ever allows us to be tempted by more than we can stand, but He will provide a way out of such temptations.**

Remember, **the Word says that WE ARE LED ASTRAY BY OUR OWN DESIRES!**

So we must SET OUR MIND that we will NOT be led astray by our own desires, KNOWING that God will not allow us to be tempted by more than we can stand, but will ALWAYS provide a way out!

Prayer: Holy Father, in the name of Jesus, I humble myself before You, knowing that I cannot, cannot, cannot fully follow The A.N.G.E.L. Plan© *without Your help, Your guidance, and Your Word. I have tried so many, many times to conquer food addiction on my own, with no success. Help me never to "diet" again, but to help me accept and embrace* The

A.N.G.E.L. Plan© *as desperately as a drowning man reaches for a life preserver!*

I pray and fast today for:

____

____

____

In the name of Jesus! Amen and amen. Selah.

13

For God has not given us a spirit of fear and timidity,
but of power and love and a sound mind
self-discipline and self-control.
(*2 Timothy 1:7 AMP*)

Take a few moments to meditate on each of the following questions and even write them down. It's only when we identify our fears for what they are that we can move into a place where we can let those fears go and let FAITH rise up instead…

First, are you afraid to look at what you're afraid of?

Are you afraid to lose weight?

Are you afraid of being more attractive?

Are you afraid to give up the "dance with diets" and counting calories and fats and carbs?

Are you actually afraid of being more beautiful?

Are you afraid to fast?

Are you afraid you won't make it and you'll be discouraged all over again?

Are you afraid you're not strong enough?

The key—the ONLY key—is to allow God to direct our fasting and eating; His Word and His Holy Spirit is OUR STRENGTH AND OUR HOPE!

We are not given a spirit of fear, but **at the moment of salvation, we receive the seeds of ALL the fruits of the Spirit—including a sound mind, self-discipline, and self-control.**

*Prayer: Father, no matter what time of day it is, help me to remember that I MUST ALLOW THE HOLY SPIRIT TO GIVE ME YOUR STRENGTH—and to **RELY on the fruit of Your Spirit of self-discipline and self-control.***

*Dear Father, in the name of Jesus, please let me live and eat in accordance with Your will—**You are my ONLY HOPE!** I love You and* *praise You and thank You, Father, that I am walking and living and eating in Your strength, control, and discipline and* **in the power of the name of Jesus!**

I pray and fast today for:

____

____

____

Amen.

14

*For the weapons of our warfare
are not carnal,
but mighty through God
to the pulling down of strongholds.
Casting down imaginations,
and every high thing that exalts itself
against the knowledge of God
and bringing into captivity
every thought to the obedience of Christ....*
(2 Corinthians 10:4–5 KJ21)

It is so wonderful to wake up knowing that God has you! He's got your back. Angels are assigned to watch over and battle the enemy for you. The Holy Ghost of Jesus Christ lives and moves within you. You only must reach within yourself and let the Holy Spirit rise up and take over your steps, your actions, your reactions, your thoughts, your words, and your fasting!

God says the weapons of our warfare are not physical or tangible, but they are spiritual and mighty through God! We have angels assigned to us, and we must put on the whole armor of God, and we already have all the seeds of fruit of the Spirit within us—including a sound mind, self-control, and self-discipline!

We have

1) the **helmet of salvation** to protect our mind and thoughts;
2) the **breastplate of righteousness** (because we ARE the righteousness of God in Christ);
3) the **sword of the Spirit, which is the Word of God;**
4) the **belt of truth** over our entire body and mind; and
5) feet shod to spread the **gospel of peace**....

Put them all on! Focus, as best you can, on each piece of armor, one at a time as you take up your spiritual weapons of warfare every morning!

Prayer: Dear God, my Holy Father, Lord Jesus, mighty Holy Ghost, in the name of Jesus I pray that You will manifest the fruits of the Spirit in me daily, including a sound mind, self-control, and self-discipline during the times that I fast OR feast. Give me Your strength, please, when I'm tempted to overeat during the times when I don't fast.

My Lord, help me to resist all the temptations of satan and his demons and little minions when they show their ugly faces—in commercials, advertisements, or offerings of food or sweets from others!

I pray and fast today for:

____

____

____

In the name of Jesus, help me, Father, because I can do nothing if I don't have the strength that only comes from You! In the name of Jesus, amen!

15

*For **the weapons of our warfare are not physical** [weapons of flesh and blood], but **they are mighty before God for the overthrow and destruction of strongholds** (areas where satan consistently attacks our minds).*

*[Inasmuch as we] **refute arguments and theories and reasonings and every proud and lofty thing that sets itself up against the [true] knowledge of God; and we lead every thought and purpose away captive into the obedience of Christ (the Messiah, the Anointed One).***
(2 Corinthians 10:4–5 AMP)

Our own mind is a dangerous place to go and play alone. satan and all his demons and evil spirits and little minions will attack and mess with our minds when we allow our mind to go where it wants…

We must cast down evil and negative thoughts, bind them in the name of Jesus, and teach ourselves to bring every thought, idea, word, expression, every emotion, and our stubborn will into captivity to the obedience of Jesus Christ.

God did not say you're a failure, and there's no hope for you! **God did say that He is more than enough to meet every trial and temptation**, that we can cast down all negative and evil and selfish thoughts in the name of Jesus. He has given you authority and power over the enemy!

It is only when we can bring our mind, our thoughts, our will, our emotions, our words, our expressions, and our actions into captivity to the obedience of Jesus Christ that we can move forward into the life He died to give us (2 Corinthians 10:4–5 KJV)! Praise and gratitude is the key to tapping into His joy and strength and victory!

Prayer: Holy Father, in the precious, glorious, and mighty name of Jesus, forgive me of my sins and negativity and doubt. **Help me, please, Lord, to bring my mind, thoughts, emotions, words, expressions, actions, and my very will into captivity to the obedience of Christ moment by moment!** *Help me… **Change me as only You can!***

I pray and fast today for:

____

____

____

In the name of Jesus, amen.

16

Do you like honey?
Don't eat too much, or it will make you sick!"…
It's not good to eat too much honey, and it's
not good to seek honors for yourself.
A person without self-control
is like a city with broken-down walls.
(Proverbs 25:16, 27–28 NLT)

The Bible gives us lots of common-sense advice about eating, and most importantly, **Jesus indicated that we are to observe a regular practice of fasting and prayer.** We are told above that it's not good to eat too much honey (or sugar and sweets) to which we all can testify—but the Word follows with *"it's not good to seek honors for yourself."*

As we begin to see our physical appearance change before our own eyes—and in the admiration of those around us—**it is so, so tempting to take credit ourselves for the blessed riddance of pounds or a healthy weight.** *We are cautioned against taking honor for ourselves instead of giving the glory to God,* **who is the author and perfector of our faith, and the true author of** *A New Godly Eating Lifestyle©.*

Verse 28 tells us that *"a person without self-control is like a city with broken-down walls."* How very well we know that statement to be true! Yet 2 Timothy 2:17 **announces to us** that *"God has not given us a spirit of fear or timidity, but of power, love, and self-discipline!"* If we are *walking in the Holy Spirit,* **we already have self-control!**

Prayer: Abba Father (my Daddy), deep down I know in my "knower" that **You have genuinely done for me and continue to do for me, what I could not and cannot do for myself. As I learn to walk in the self-discipline of the Holy Spirit, help me to submit to**

Your will and make good choices that are healthy and satisfying to me.

Thank you that I do not have to be deprived of any food, and I have the newfound freedom to fast and to eat as You will, under the discipline of the Holy Spirit.

I pray and fast today for:

____

____

____

In the holy and miraculous name of Jesus, amen!

17

No temptation has overtaken you
except such as is common to mankind.
*And **God is faithful;***
He will not let you be tempted
beyond what you can bear.
But when you are tempted,
He will also provide a way out
so that you can endure it.
(1 Corinthians 10:13 NKJV)

What a precious, lifesaving promise of God! So many times, when food seems our only "friend"—the only thing that we can control around us is something inside of us—when in truth, it is a devil's lie!

satan's only weapons are fear and deception! Don't be afraid to call it what it is—an outright lie of the enemy! **Food is not—and never has been—our comforter or friend**. It is sustenance to our body and can be thoroughly enjoyed when it is combined with intermittent fasting.

Many people will never make it this far in this devotional because their fear of failure—based on past failure keeps them from even trying, or their fear of failure sabotages their early efforts.

Jesus said,

Come to Me,
all you who labor and are heavy laden,
And I will give you rest.
Take My yoke upon you and learn from Me,
for I am gentle and lowly in heart,
and you will find rest for your souls.
For My Yoke is easy and My burden is light.
(Matthew 11:28–30 NKJV)

*Prayer: Lord Jesus, thank You that **I am right now able to cast my cares on You.** Thank You that I don't have to pull a yoke of worry, problems, and stumbling blocks alone in my yoke, but that You invite and allow me to get in Your yoke with You so **You can help me pull my load!** Thank You, Lord, that I am learning from You and **that Your yoke is easy and Your burden is light.***

I pray and fast today for:

____

____

____

Father, thank You for all Your sustaining promises, in the holy name of Jesus, amen.

18

No weapon formed against you shall prosper!
(Isaiah 54:17 NKJV)

What a promise to stand firmly on—when the darts of the enemy hit us from one side or from all sides, when stuff just keeps happening, when unexpected problems arise, like a worldwide pandemic, when we used to turn to food as a comfort or to hide, we tried to control our circumstances by ingesting whatever we wanted into our bodies to satisfy our craving for comfort and peace; yet that only worked for a moment—the rest on our hips!

We have submitted to and dedicated ourselves to *A New Godly Eating Lifestyle*©**, and as such, I can firmly stand on the promise** that: *No weapon formed against me shall prosper!*

Recognize temptation during your dedicated fasting period for what it is—temptation by the devil—and we are also led astray by our own desires and lusts…to keep us from the benefits and blessings of *A New Godly Eating Lifestyle*©· Then **we can draw on the power of the Holy Spirit within us and the fruit of self-discipline.** The more often we do this, the sooner resisting temptation becomes second nature to us, and we can discern through the Spirit what we genuinely want or need to eat. You will find that your appetite is changing, and when it's time to eat, you want good healthy food.

Remember, the only rule is, **there is a time to fast and a time to feast. We must learn the difference and it's all about the timing. It's not WHAT you eat nearly as much as it is WHEN you eat!**

Fasting or feasting—lots and lots of our Living Water and more water, water, water….

Prayer: Our awesome maker, our Living Water—the Creator of all things, ***thank You that no weapon, even weapons of my own devise, that are formed against me shall prosper nor succeed in any way!***

Thank You that You allow no temptation beyond what I am able to stand, and that You always provide a way out!

Help those of my fellows who have chosen **A New Godly Eating Lifestyle,** *as we walk the path toward healthy living and feeling and looking the best we can, but only for Your glory, honor, and praise!*

I pray and fast today for:

____

____

____

In Jesus's holy name, amen.

19

But Jesus beheld them and said unto them,
"With men, this is impossible,
but with God all things are possible!"
(Matthew 19:23 KJV)

How often we've heard this scripture, but do we really believe it? **Do YOU really believe it? Pause** to look inside yourself and answer that question **now**.

If you don't believe it, ask Jesus to "author" within you a firm and deepening faith, since the Bible declares He is the author and the finisher (the perfector) of our faith. As you continue to pray this, you will find that your faith to believe that all things are possible with God is growing increasingly stronger, and you can then ask Jesus to "finish" or "perfect" your faith, so that you may stand firm in His promises to the finish line.

You may still find it hard to believe that following *The A.N.G.E.L. Plan*© will give you a complete freedom over the enslavement to food and that you'll have an amazing body in its healthy and correct size. You may not think it possible that *The A.N.G.E.L. Plan*© will correct a hypoactive thyroid, but it does! Proof is in the bloodwork! See "My Freedom Story" in chapter 6.

"With men, this is impossible, but with God all
things are possible!" (Matthew 19:23 NKJV).

Prayer: Lord Jesus, You are the author and finisher and perfector of my faith. Increase and deepen my faith, Lord, as I linger and walk daily in Your presence and learn of You. ***Lord, please author within me the true deep-seated belief that with You and God all things are possible!***

I pray and fast today for:

____

____

____

It is more than possible that I shall follow The A.N.G.E.L. Plan©
to health, restoration, and a healthier body, and no longer be encumbered
by the guilt and weight of gluttonous sin, in the name of Jesus! Amen.

20

Then Jesus said,
"Come to Me, all of you who are weary
and carry heavy burdens, and I will give you rest.
Take My yoke upon you. Let Me teach you,
because I am humble and gentle at heart,
and you will find rest for your souls.
"For My yoke is easy to bear,
and the burden I give you is light."
(Matthew 11:28–30 NLT)

The constant burden, the nagging thoughts, the guilt, remorse, frustration, and even self-hatred are almost unbearable for the one addicted to food.

Jesus said we didn't have to do that struggle alone, and we've prayed and prayed and prayed. Yet so few of us obey the commands of the Word of God and Jesus regarding prayer and fasting.

Giving ourselves to *The A.N.G.E.L. Plan*© will be frustrating and even difficult the first three or four days, but very easily you'll transition into eating good foods when hungry to get what your body tells you that you need. (Chocolate is not a need!) You'll begin to "eat to live, rather than living to eat."

Jesus wants you **out of your yoke of bondage to food,** and He invites you to join Him in His yoke, which is easy to bear and a much, much lighter burden. **YOU take the first step to get in the yoke with Jesus, and He'll carry you forward into victory!**

Prayer: Jehovah Jirah! Our provider!
In the name of Jesus, we bless and praise and glorify and thank You for the successes we continue to have every day that we adhere to The A.N.G.E.L. Plan©*! May we never take credit for our victory.*
Let me share that it is Your Word that sets us free, through intermittent fasting, continual prayer and water!

I pray and fast today for:

____

____

____

We commit today and every day to You, to follow Your lead and direction every step of the way, and we THANK YOU, FATHER, IN THE NAME OF JESUS! Amen.

21

Wait patiently for the Lord.
Be brave and courageous.
Yes, wait patiently for the Lord.
(Psalm 27:14 NLT)

Oh, if we could only learn the lessons God brings into our lives in an instant, rather than over days and weeks and months and years....

I was especially hardheaded about trying to hurry God along. I still even try to do it! Yet God will not be hurried. He has a perfect plan, with perfect timing, and it will come to fruition in His own perfect time.

No one really wants to pray for patience because it seems to always bring on trials and tests of our faith. However, there are great rewards!

James exhorts us in James 1:2–4 (NKJV):

My brethren, count it all Joy
when you fall into various trials,
knowing that the testing of your Faith
produces Patience.
But let Patience have its perfect work,
that you may be perfect and complete,
lacking nothing.

WOW! WHAT A PROMISE!

Prayer: Father, as we are growing in the fruit of the spirit of patience, help us to surrender to the Holy Spirit, letting "self" go.... Please remind me, Lord, that trials will always test our faith, and the testing of our faith in You produces patience and many other fruits of Your Spirit!

I pray and fast today for:

____

____

____

I thank You that patience is having its perfect work in me that I may be perfect and complete, lacking nothing! In the name of Jesus, amen!

22

A peaceful heart leads to a healthy body;
jealousy is like cancer in the bones.
(*Proverbs 14:30 NLT*)

By the time we come to this meditation, we have all experienced unrest in our souls about our eating, our weight, our body, our image, guilt at using food to distort our bodies, guilt at our secret eating, even guilt at "overeating" during our committed fasting times. Let the guilt go! This is a lifestyle—not a diet that you can break!

A main goal of *The A.N.G.E.L. Plan*© is to find PEACE within ourselves regarding food, meals, snacks, and our harmful eating habits in general. We do that by releasing the guilt of man's expectations for our eating and grasping the life preserver of the Word of God, which points us to health and inward peace toward food—**prayer and fasting.**

While the Old Testament believers practiced fasting, many Christians act like that is no longer expected of us. Yet in the New Testament, Jesus said, **"When you fast…." He didn't say IF you fast—He said WHEN you fast. He expects it from us. He has ordained prayer and fasting for healing of the body.**

Our verse today includes peace and the very next subject is jealousy. We have all known jealousy in one form or another, whether jealousy of what another person has or looks like, or jealousy of your significant other with other people. Our minds can literally run wild! satan loves to cause jealousy, so recognize the enemy for what he is!

Resist the urge to eat back at them (or smoke or drink at them!)

Only God can take away the jealousy—LET HIM! SUR-RENDER the jealousy—or it will literally eat you up… like cancer in the bones.

In 1 Corinthians 13, the apostle Paul expounds on the meaning of love. In verses 4–5, he tells us:

Love is patient and kind.
Love is not jealous or boastful or proud or rude.
It does not demand its own way.
It is not irritable and keeps no record of being wronged.

When we are jealous, we are not walking in complete love. We need to search ourselves and ask God to help us determine the root cause of our jealousy—no matter what or how many kinds—and to give us the wisdom to deal with it and to let God cut jealousy out at the core.

Prayer: Father, in the holy and precious name of Jesus, hear my cry, oh Lord! Please just help me. **Help me in the way You know I need. Please reveal to me the reasons why I choose to turn to food—instead of turning to YOU, Lord God. I ask that You take away jealousy in every form within me and** *help me please to* **find REST in YOU in my heart and soul, in my mind, my will, my thoughts, and my emotions.**

I pray and fast today for:

____

____

____

I thank You that You have already answered my prayers and my answers are coming into fruition on this earthly plain, in the name of Jesus!

23

*Keep watch and pray,
so that you will not give in
to temptation.
For the spirit is willing,
but the body is weak!*
(Matthew 26:41 NLT)

One of the most important exhortations that Jesus gave to His disciples is to **"Keep watch"** and to "**pray so that you will not give in to temptation."**

Temptation *NEVER, EVER* comes from God! Temptation is all satan's doing. **The Lord said that we are led astray by our own lusts and desires.** Moreover, the Word says that **God will never tempt us, but with each temptation, He will give us a way out, and that He will NOT allow us to be tempted beyond that which we can stand.**

It is so vitally important that as we continue in *A New Godly Eating Lifestyle*© that **we start each day with prayer, bringing our mind, thoughts, will, emotions, words, and expressions into captivity to the obedience of Christ (2 Corinthians 10:4–5 KJV). We must submit ourselves to God early in our day and continually throughout our day and night**, THANKING GOD **for each moment of success that we achieve that day through His strength and power!**

Prayer: **Father, in Jesus's precious name, I submit my mind, thoughts, will, emotions, words, and expressions into captivity to the obedience of Christ.** *Please help me every step of the way because I know deep down in my inner core that **I cannot bear this journey of life or* The A.N.G.E.L. Plan© *without Your help.***

I pray, dear Father, that I will not give in to temptation for I know that my Spirit is willing but my body is weak.

I pray and fast today for:

____

____

____

Thank You for all that You are! Amen.

24

I am the Bread of Life.
Whoever comes to Me
will never be hungry again.
Whoever believes in Me
will never be thirsty.
(John 6:35 NLT)

Imagine that! It is possible that we should never hunger or thirst again—only as we REST in CHRIST.

Getting to that place of rest in Christ takes time and practice. Yes, practice! Practice telling yourself that you are resting in God and turning over even the smallest problem or obstruction or adversity to Him Who created each one of us.

Practice realizing and actually experiencing **HIS GREAT LOVE FOR YOU** to the greatest degree possible. It's often difficult to realize God's intense and never-ending Love for us when we do not fully love ourselves for one reason or another—or from one moment to another.

As we have learned to lean on Him daily, hourly, moment by moment, and to find rest in Him and experience His eternal Love for us, then we become ASSURED that we can handle any period of fasting that He calls us to do, whether daily, hourly, momentarily—and then weekly, monthly, and annually, and time passes, and **we are literally made new in Him!**

Prayer: **Dear Father, Lord Jesus, Holy Ghost, embrace me in Your love and Your rest and take away the physical desires for excess food—food beyond my need, and help me, Lord—HELP ME, PLEASE—to be satisfied in You rather than food or drink.**

Jesus, YOU are the Bread of Life and the Living Water, *and I thank YOU over and over and over for giving me* **freedom from enslavement to worry, anxiety, stress, guilt, gluttony, and food!**

I pray and fast today for:

____

____

____

In Your precious and most holy name! Amen and amen.

25

*I can do all things through Christ
Who strengthens me!*
(Philippians 4:13 AMP)

For twenty-five days, you have successfully engaged in *A New Godly Eating Lifestyle*, whether you've done it "perfectly" or not. In a lifestyle, there is no "perfect" for the rest of your earthly life, so you can just accept that.

A diet is a diet, set for a certain period of time or for a certain goal.

A LIFESTYLE is a new way to live, to see, to approach life. Here we learn Godly eating patterns that literally CHANGE YOUR LIFE and YOUR BODY and the way you see food, temptation, and freedom.

You are learning to eat to live—no longer to live to eat! God has done this for you through your obedience to and direction of the Holy Scripture and the Holy Ghost Who lives inside of you!

You have always had this ability to surrender to the Holy Ghost, but satan has attacked your mind, will, thoughts, emotions and attitudes with selfishness, fear, guilt, and condemnation! We fear never having enough. **We fear that we will not get what we want or that we will lose what we have.** That makes us angry.

It's satan's way, those are his only tricks, and they stand USELESS when we are leaning on and resting in God to fight this battle. As Jesus said, **some (things) come out only by prayer and fasting.**

Prayer: Father, in the amazing name of Jesus, I thank You and thank You and thank You again and again for what You have done and continue to do daily in my spirit, my mind and my physical body as I adapt to A New Godly Eating Lifestyle©.

I pray and fast today for:

____

____

____

I surrender to Your Holy Spirit now and all of today, and Praise and Honor YOUR glorious name, oh, God, in the name of Jesus!

26

Ye are of God, little children, and have overcome…
*Because **Greater is He that is in you***
than he that is in the world.
(1 John 4:4 KJV)

The Lord is my strength and my shield.
I trust Him with all my heart!
He helps me, and
my heart is filled with joy.
I burst out in songs of thanksgiving!
(Psalms 28:7 NLT)

What comfort this verse brings to me! Especially when I'm feeling negative and hopeless on so many fronts.

WE ARE OF GOD—and because WE ARE OF GOD, then we have the fruits of the Holy Spirit evidenced in our lives and witness, AND the seeds of the fruits of the Spirit were given to us at the moment we accepted Jesus as Lord and Master and Savior—and those fruits include **self-control and self-discipline.**

Those seeds of the fruits of the Spirit are already inside of you—we just have to learn to tap into and lean in and develop them through seeking God in fasting, prayer, teachings, and meditation on the Words of God.

Imagine that—and then begin to feel the fruits of the Spirit in your inward soul—your mind, will, thoughts, emotions, expressions, and expectations!

Prayer: My Lord God Almighty, Worthy is Your name to be praised throughout the heavens and throughout the earth! satan flees at the mention of Your name, Lord Jesus! You are omniscient, omnipresent, all-knowing, all-powerful, and ALL LOVE!

Thank you, Father, that we are Your "little children" and You have empowered us, moment by moment, to overcome any temptation or fiery darts of the devil and to STAND STRONG and REST IN YOU.
I pray and fast today for:

____

____

____

In the name of Jesus, amen!

27

*That is why **I tell you not to worry**
about everyday life—
Whether you have enough food and drink,
or enough clothes to wear.
"Isn't life more than food,
and your body more than clothing?"
(Matthew 6:25 NLT)*

What are our basic physical needs in the natural world? First, we look for shelter, and our next concern is for protection (who will protect us from the enemies immediate or future?). Then we seek water to drink, food to eat, and clothes to wear for cover.

By now, you've learned some basic principles about how **God always, always, always, always provides those things which we need**. If the next steps in front of us are uncertain or we just can't understand the reasons for what lies before us, **we KNOW that God will provide those needs and answers for us. We don't trust in only the things which we can see tangibly or immediately ahead, but we trust that GOD has ways of meeting ALL our needs—** His perfect place of shelter and protection, our drink, our food, our clothes—**day by day and moment by moment.**

Once we realize that God's timing is NOT necessarily our timing, but that His timing is perfect, then we can relax and rest in and TRUST IN GOD to handle any and every situation or fiery dart or temptation of the enemy.

*Prayer: Abba Father, in the most holy name of Jesus, let my prayer today be that of **thanksgiving, praise, and joy** that You've brought me this far—farther than I ever knew possible—and I will continue to **stay** in close fellowship with You to enjoy worship, praise, thanksgiving, joy, as well as healing in my body and health to my bones!*

I thank You today that my **every single need has already been met, every prayer answered, and I have only to receive it with a grateful heart.**

I pray and fast today for:

____

____

____

In the precious name of Jesus I pray, amen.

28

He said to them,
"I have food to eat of which you do not know."
Therefore, the disciples said to one another,
"Has anyone brought Him anything to eat?"
Jesus said to them,
"My food is to do the will of Him
Who sent Me, and to finish His work."
(John 4:32–34 NKJV)

Jesus taught us this: ***"I am the Bread of Life. He who comes to Me will never be hungry, and he who believes in and cleaves to and trusts in and relies on Me will never thirst anymore"*** (John 6:35 AMPC).

Jesus also proclaimed that **HIS FOOD was to do the will of God Who sent Him! It is food to our bodies to do the will of God.** Food was intended to satisfy our physical hunger, and that is all! **Food was not intended by God to be a fortress or a shelter or a refuge or a "hiding place."** Taking our feelings and emotions and anger and frustration to FOOD is quite useless!

Moreover, it is taking our problems and boredom to FOOD instead of taking them to GOD.

God's first commandment is ***"You shall have no other gods before or besides me"*** (Exodus 20:3 AMPC).

Question: **Am I putting food before God's will in my priorities?**

While we go through our committed fasting period, we do well to remind ourselves when we feel either physical or emotional "hunger pangs or pains" to ***turn to God in Christ, Who gives us our strength!*** **We can do all things through Christ who gives us strength!** (Philippians 4:13).

*Prayer: Thank You, Jesus, our Almighty Father and my **inner Holy Ghost!** Thank You that **I can do all things that I need to do to accomplish Your will through Your strength and power, Lord Jesus!***

I pray and fast today for:

____

____

____

Thank you that YOU and Your will are my priority over resorting to food for anything other than relief of hunger! In the name of Jesus, *amen and amen.*

29

My eyes are always on the Lord,
for He rescues me from the traps of my enemies.
(*Psalm 25:15 NLT*)

One thing I know for certain is that **God's love never fails me!**

As you completely devote yourself to *A New Godly Eating Lifestyle©*, **after you first seek God's will in all you do, and as you dedicate your times of fasting to God**—you will find that you love God far more than you did before and that you are learning to love **yourself!** You can fast to achieve weight loss, or fast for a relationship, or fast for healing—whatever you are seeking God about—and **dedicate yourself to learning more of God and knowing Him and** loving Him back as much as He loves you!

TAKE A FEW MINUTES JUST TO WORSHIP THE FATHER, THE SON, AND THE HOLY GHOST who dwells inside you to give you strength!

THE POWER OF PRAISE AND WORSHIP, THE POWER OF GRATITUDE, AND THE POWER OF PRAYER AND FASTING CANNOT POSSIBLY BE OVERSTATED!

You will find that as you learn to trust in and rely on God and LOVE GOD BACK that you will begin to love YOURSELF in a far greater way than you ever have before, and *you will experience peace and joy like you never knew possible!*

For God's sake! Yes, "for the sake of seeking God"—as well as your own sake and your loved ones' sake—**allow yourself to submit to, relax in, trust in, and obey the Word and spiritual laws of the Lord regarding life and also toward food and drink.** You'll begin to actually look forward to and really enjoy *A New Godly Eating Lifestyle©*.

You WILL fully know freedom from enslavement to gluttony and that never-ending battle with food!

Prayer: Father God, thank You that You are ALL to me! Your holiness brings me to my face on the ground, yet I know that as my "Daddy" I can rest my head in Your lap, dear Lord.

I pray and fast today for:

____

____

____

I thank You that You knew what I needed—and provision was already on the way before *I knew I needed it!*

Thank You that today miracles will happen to me as I thank and praise my way through my day, loving You back with all my heart and soul and mind—in the name of Jesus! Amen.

30

Behold, God is my salvation,
I will trust and not be afraid;
For Yay, the Lord, is my strength and song;
He also has become my salvation...
Praise the Lord,
Call upon His name;
Declare His deeds among the peoples,
Make mention that His name is exalted.
Sing to the Lord,
For He has done excellent things;
This is known in all the earth.
(Isaiah 12:2–5 NKJV)

What excellent verses of scripture! I must open my mouth to sing and praise and call upon Him! I must declare His deeds among the people and make mention that His name be exalted!

Instead of using my mouth to complain or backbite or gossip, **I must be transformed by the renewing of my mind through the Word of God!**

Praise and gratitude, peace and the joy of the Lord always leave us "feeling full" of the Holy Spirit! I must submit my mouth to God, resist the devil and he will flee from me.

During your fasting period when you get hungry, let the joy of the Lord be your strength and your song. Drink a glass of water or more, which will curb those hunger pangs. When you feel them, sow those hunger pangs into the focus of your fast that day. Commit those hunger pangs to God, and what we do in secret He rewards openly!

Prayer: Father, I thank You and praise You and glorify Your name throughout the earth! Thank you that Your joy is my strength and my song, and help me to speak positive, lovely, and beautiful words of hope and faith throughout the day.

I pray and fast today for:

____

____

____

In the name of Jesus, amen.

31

And He, bearing His cross, went out to
a place called the Place of a Skull,
which is called in Hebrew, Golgotha,
where they crucified Him,
and two others with Him....
He said, "It is Finished!"
And bowing His head,
He gave up His Spirit.
(John 19:17–18, 30 NKJV)

Jesus paid the ultimate price and presented the perfect offering for the sins of all mankind so that He could present us to the Father washed clean and as white as snow through His shed blood on the cross, **with no remnant of sin remaining in us.** When we receive Him as our personal savior, begging forgiveness, and being thankful and worshipful at all times according to His grace working in us, then we begin to grow in the fruits of the Holy Spirit. **At salvation, we receive the seeds of all of the fruits of the Spirit, which are love, joy, peace, patience, kindness, faithfulness, gentleness, and self-control** (Galatians 5:22 NKJV).

God leads us through the navigation of life through both His blessings and the troubles that satan brings into our lives. In these ways, He begins to reveal, and we begin to grow in, the fruits of the Spirit in us. **As we learn MORE OF HIM, the quicker our fruits of the Spirit will grow and the healthier we become.**

The more we grow in self-control, self-discipline, and soundness of mind, **the easier it is to pass up** treats or eating during your fasting period. It actually does become easy! You will hardly be able to believe it!

Prayer: Holy Father, I humbly acknowledge and accept Christ's gift on the cross and take you again as my Lord, Master, and Savior. Help me to seek and receive the fruits of the Spirit, which includes self-control.

I pray and fast today for:

____

____

____

Help me, Lord, as I continue with A NEW GODLY EATING LIFESTYLE©, *to learn* MORE OF YOU *as You help make my crooked places straight, as I seek the fruit of self-control to defeat the devil in the food temptations he places before me. In the holy, precious and powerful name of Jesus, amen and amen.*

32

Coming out, He went to the Mount of Olives,
as He was accustomed, and
His disciples also followed Him.
When He came to the place, He said to them,
"Pray that you may not enter into temptation."
And He was withdrawn from them, about a stone's throw,
and He knelt down and prayed, saying,
"Father, if it is Your will,
take this cup from Me;
nevertheless, not my will, but Yours, be done."
Then an angel appeared from Heaven,
strengthening Him.
(Luke 22:39–43 NKJV)

Jesus was so very tempted in the Garden of Gethsemane to use His omnipotent power to escape the crucifixion before Him, taking on all human sins throughout infinity. Jesus went to prayer three separate times seeking God's mercy to avoid crucifixion on a cross. He was in such agony that He shed **sweat drops of blood!** (Luke 22:44 NKJV).

We face daily temptations of all kinds of vices and bad behavior, ***including eating "fancy food."***

We are sometimes tempted to skip our morning praise and worship, meditation, and daily devotions of *The A.N.G.E.L. Plan©* or to skip our actual prayers, Bible study, specific petitions. Not only are we tempted to skip our morning devotions, but we may simply forget to **THANK AND PRAISE HIM for our answers that we already have and those which are already on the way!**

That is one of our biggest pitfalls every day—failing to pray and failing to commit to our *A.N.G.E.L. Plan©*.

Jesus clearly instructed us Matthew 26:41 (NKJV) to, **"Watch and pray, lest you enter into temptation. The Spirit is indeed willing but the flesh is weak."**

Prayer:** Holy Father, in the name of Jesus, we THANK YOU that You have promised that **You will always provide a way out of temptation if we will resist the desires of the flesh!

I want to THANK YOU for all others entering into A New Godly Eating Lifestyle©, and I ask You to strengthen them and teach them a new way of living also!

I pray and fast today for:

____

____

____

Please give us wisdom and knowledge, dear Lord, especially during our times of eating, *so that we may keep our temples healthy and become more glorified by You in this present world. Amen.*

33

*Enter into His gates with Thanksgiving, and
into His courts with praise!
Be thankful to Him and bless His name.*
(Psalm 100:4 NKJV)

Throughout the time I've been writing *The A.N.G.E.L. Plan*©, I have learned that the most important part of my prayer time is GIVING THANKS for all things in my life, including the tiniest of things **and** the trials I go through.

Gratitude to God is one of the most important privileges and traits that we can incorporate into our lives. Sometimes, like when I'm not feeling well or am just upset, I have to ask God to put gratitude in my heart toward Him, and also toward the others whose path I cross. And He does.

Psalm 100:4 above strongly tells us to **"enter His courts with praise!"** My best prayer time is when I come boldly before God's throne in the name of Jesus and give Him both thanks **and** praise! **God inhabits the praises of His people**.

More specifically, we are to, **"Rejoice always, pray without ceasing, give thanks in all circumstances, because this is the will of God in Christ Jesus" for you** (1 Thessalonians 5:16–18 NKJV).

In *A New Godly Eating Lifestyle*©, we are grateful for the food we eat during our eating times, and soon we desire healthy "real" food, rather than sweets and carbs.

*Prayer: Abba Father, we **thank You and praise You and glorify You for all of Your mighty works, down to the smallest atom in our bodies.** You are mighty and worthy to be praised **every day, all day** as we are led to pray without ceasing.*

I pray and fast today for:

____

____

____

Thank you, holy God, for giving us the strength to change our **entire lifestyle** *through Your divine inspiration, in the name of Jesus we pray, amen.*

34

But when you fast, anoint your head and wash your face, that your fasting may not be seen by others but by your Father who is in secret. And your Father who sees in secret will reward you. *(Matthew 6:17–18 ESV)*

In His Sermon on the Mount (Matthew 5–7), Jesus taught us, among other things, too fast. He told us that what we should **not do** is make a big display of denying ourselves and let others know we are fasting. All glory goes to God!

However, Jesus **promised** that if we wash our face, anoint our head, and fast in secret, that **"your Father who sees in secret *will reward you*!"** In the same way we are to go into our room (closet) and seek God and pray privately so as not to be seen by others.

When a person fasts, they are generally seeking some kind of reward. It could be as simple as a fast to enable them to grow in a particular fruit of the Spirit, or to save a nation as Esther did, or for weight loss or for healing a thyroid. We often fast for the salvation or healing of a loved one, a spouse, a child, a friend, a marriage, for restoration or to beat depression.

I believe that whomever or whatever is on your heart that morning is what you might seek from God during your fasting periods. You can fast for several things. You fast for what is on *your* heart. God knows our hearts, and "Father knows best."

As we see progress in ourselves, whether in our spirit or in our body, we have much to **GIVE THANKS AND PRAISE TO GOD** about and to celebrate our progress! (Not necessarily a chocolate or carb binge!)

Be careful that as you look healthier and thinner (if that is your goal) that you don't take praise or pride in yourself, but that you give God the praise and thanks that He so richly and rightfully deserves!

Prayer: Lord God Jehovah! Jehovah Jirah! I know that You see my fasting, whether done secretly or publicly if necessary. **Your Word promises that the fasting I do in secret You will reward!**

I pray and fast today for:

____

____

____

Jesus, You are our Living Water and our daily Bread of Life. *Thank You that You have enabled and anointed me to immerse myself into* A New Godly Eating Lifestyle© *and that I am reaping Your promised rewards. In Your holy name I pray, amen.*

35

For in it the righteousness of God
is revealed from faith to faith,
as it is written,
"The just shall live by faith."
(Romans 1:17 NKJV)

Faith must be stirred up within you and released. When it seems we have no faith, we can ask Jesus to "author" in us a deeper faith and that He "finish" or "perfect" our faith.

*Looking unto **Jesus,**
the author and finisher
of our faith,
who for the joy set before Him
endured the cross,
despising the shame, and has **sat**
down on the right hand
at the throne of God.
(Hebrews 12:2 NKJV)*

We release our faith by praying, speaking of the present as if answers have already come, and letting our actions show that we are moving forward to that destination.

Prayer: *Thank You, Holy Father, that I feel alive again, more in touch with my true self! I know through* A New Godly Eating Lifestyle© *that I am learning that my body and myself are not the same. I know now that food is only fuel for this body which is Your temple. I know that what I feed my spirit and soul during fasting times gives me strength to learn how to eat well and become the right body size for me.*

I pray and fast today for:

____

____

____

I pray in the holy name of Jesus, amen and amen.

36

*For no matter how many
promises God has made,
they are "Yes" in Christ.
And so through Him
the "Amen" is spoken by us
to the glory of God.*
(2 Corinthians 1:20 NIV)

God has made thousands of promises throughout the Bible. If we were to **list just the promises that we know** (not necessarily that we've memorized), we could certainly write down many of those promises even without referring to the Bible. Try it! How many promises do you know and depend on without even thinking?

God promises day and night will continue. God promises us not to destroy the earth by water again. God promises us that He will never leave us or forsake us. God promises that we can have eternal life through true belief in Jesus Christ our Lord!

God promises us that we can have a spirit of power, love, and a sound mind (self-discipline and self-control)! The fruits of the Spirit will grow in us as we seek Him, praise, thank and honor Him, and set our minds on things above, which are eternal.

Embracing *The A.N.G.E.L. Plan©: A New Godly Eating Lifestyle©*, **we quickly learn that we can and must depend on the Holy Spirit, the name of Jesus, and God our Father to provide a way out of temptations** from satan or from our own fleshly desires.

Temptation can come even through our dearest loved ones, our spouse, our best friends, our parents, our children, our siblings....

*Let no one say when he is tempted,
"I am tempted by God";
for God cannot be tempted by evil,
neither does He Himself tempt anyone.*

But each one is tempted when he is
drawn away by his own
desires and enticed.
(James 1:13–14 NKJV)

Knowing fully well that Jesus instructed us to fast in secret, I find it most helpful to let the people you live with know in general that you will be changing your eating lifestyle, and that The A.N.G.E.L. Plan© is a day-by-day lifestyle, that you can attune it for each particular day.

Prayer: *Dear Father, in the most mighty and highly exalted name of Jesus, I thank You* **for all You have done and continue to do for me** *moment by moment! I praise Your glorious name above all! Let my life be an honor to You, Lord, and show me the path you want me to take today, please. Guide me with Your eye.*

I pray and fast today for:

____

____

____

Help me, Lord, to grow in the fruits of the spirit of self-control and self-discipline so that I might easily follow The A.N.G.E.L. Plan©. *God, You said You would always provide a way out of temptation for me. Lord, please let me seek Your escape so that I might fully follow* A New Godly Eating Lifestyle—The A.N.G.E.L. Plan©. *Amen!*

37

*You do not have
because you do not ask.
You ask and do not receive,
because you ask wrongly,
to you may spend it on your
passions.*
(James 4:2–3 NIV)

In the first verse above, James tells us that if we do not properly ask God for something, we are not going to get what we have asked for. He goes on to explain that many people ask for those "things" that will thrill their flesh and fulfill all its pleasures, instead of those things that further the Gospel (Good News) of Christ and the kingdom of God.

How do we **not** pray in the flesh? By seeking first the kingdom of God and His righteousness, all these "things" will be given us.

Sometimes, our faith is so weak that it nearly fails us. It is then that we ask Jesus, the author and finisher of our faith, **to author new and abundant faith in our hearts, and then ask Him to *finish or perfect our faith*** so we can believe fully in God's promises.

Prayer: Jesus, I come to you as humbly and as gratefully as I can be now, in Your own precious name above all names, and I ask that You author within me a fresh, new faith that I may fully believe Your promises. Secondly, Jesus, I ask that you perfect my faith so my faith may be full until I see God's promises in my life. I praise and thank You that You hear me when I pray!

I pray and fast today for:

____

____

____

Lord, as I embrace A New Godly Eating Lifestyle©, *help me and all others embracing* The A.N.G.E.L. Plan© *to soar past unhealthy food or temptations of food during our fasting period. We pray also, God, for wisdom and knowledge from You regarding* The A.N.G.E.L. Plan© *that we may be self-disciplined and recognize temptations, submit ourselves to God, and resist the temptations of the enemy at once. In the name of Jesus, amen.*

38

For this reason I am telling you,
whatever things you ask for in prayer
[in accordance with God's will],
believe** [with confident trust] **that
you have received them,
and they will be given to you.
(Mark 11:24 AMP)

Prayer is the most important thing we can do each morning to start on God's path for our day. Otherwise, we may just be wondering and wandering aimlessly to figure out what we need or want to do daily.

Jesus said, **"Whatever things you ask for in prayer, believe that you have received them, and they will be given to you."** Yes, that sounds absolutely wonderful! But once again, we may come to a place where our faith may be weak or low, and fear has entered our mind and soul, making God's promises **seem** impossible. Again (and again and again and again), we can **ask Jesus to author in us the faith we need and to perfect that faith** so that we may fully know God's will for us and be fully able to receive the promises that God gave us through Jesus Christ.

KNOW in the deepest part of your mind and spirit that YOU will fully adopt *A New Godly Eating Lifestyle*© and know better health and body weight, and you may also see changes in your expectations of yourself and others.

Remember, hunger pangs will not kill you! Drink some water until those hunger pangs are gone. Hunger pangs **will** go away in a few minutes. During those hunger pangs, that is when I turn to God and pray with supplication (specifically) for whatever I am fasting about that day. Soon, this will become as easy and as natural for you as it did for me.

Prayer: Father, please help us through the hunger pangs when we are fasting so that we can know the **pure JOY of living with freedom from enslavement to food, thoughts of food, fantasizing about "fancy foods" or snacks.**

Help us to fast as Jesus instructed us so that we may more fully know You, oh God! **We pray that any "demons" of satan, through addictions, sins or weaknesses, all come out through our prayer and fasting, as You promised, Lord.**

I pray and fast today for:

____

____

____

Please keep us on the narrow road without detours, God, that You may direct our path, guide us with Your eye, and make our crooked places straight. In the name of Jesus, amen and amen.

39

**No temptation has overtaken you
except such as is common to man.
And GOD IS FAITHFUL:
He will not let you be
tempted beyond what you can bear.
But when you are tempted, He will also
provide a way out so that you can endure it.**
(1 Corinthians 10:13 NIV)

This scripture is **so very comforting** as we embrace our *New Godly Eating Lifestyle*©. Most of us are tempted to eat too much, or we may be tempted to not eat at all to stay skinny.

That is why our full dependence on God, to help us through temptation and to find a way out of it, is critical for everyone.

These devotions are intended to strengthen you and remind you how easy it is to fully submit to *The A.N.G.E.L. Plan*© after the first three or four days. I want to share with you how critical it is that we first seek God in our day as soon as we awaken. **Your JOY can be full!**

*Prayer: THANK YOU, Father God, that **You are always faithful to me**! I thank You that You will not let me be tempted beyond what I can stand, and that when I am tempted that **You "always provide a way out so that I can endure it."***

I pray and fast today for:

____

____

____

Thank you, Lord, that I am experiencing the effects of The A.N.G.E.L. Plan© *in my mind and my body, and that all **glory and honor belong to You, Father,** and not to me! In the name of Jesus, amen.*

40

Beloved, I pray that in every way
you may prosper in all things
and be in health,
just as your soul prospers.
(3 John 1:2 NKJV)

I love this verse, especially since I truly dedicated my life to Jesus Christ. Fortunately, God has given me a hunger for His Word and the teaching of His Word such that there's nothing I'd rather do first thing in the morning than to spend several hours with Him, learning of Him, growing in Him, leaning on Him, talking to Him and most importantly, listening to Him.

This verse gives us HOPE. As we put God first in all things and really seek to KNOW HIM, He will cause us to prosper and be in good health in accordance with the way our soul prospers.

As I keep GOD FIRST in all things, I find that the nagging thoughts of food (eating it, passing it up, cooking it, preserving it, tossing it) **are not present anymore.** I usually don't crave that dessert after dinner.

When I end my fast, I want *healthy* food instead of carbs and sweets. *I have the freedom to eat any of those, but I find my appetite has rapidly changed.*

God promises us that He will never allow us to be tempted beyond what we are able to stand, but He will in each situation provide a way out!

Prayer: Holy Father, I come to You in the precious and most holy name of Jesus, and I thank You and praise You for the progress I've made today. I thank You that I'm not on some fad diet, but I have fully embraced A New Godly Eating Lifestyle© *and am on my way to a more physically healthy body and freedom from the bondage of food!*

Help me, Lord, to escape temptations that come my way daily, that You may find me more pleasing to You, Father.
I pray and fast today for:

____

____

____

In the name of Jesus, amen and amen.

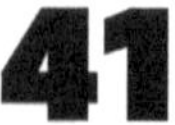

Therefore, submit to God,
resist the devil
and he will flee from you.
Draw near to God and
He will draw near to you.
(James 4:7–8 NKJV)

"Submit to God"—what does that even mean? How do I really do that?

"Submit" wasn't even in my vocabulary until I met Jesus Christ! Perhaps you've had the same questions or experience. I've tried numerous times in many ways to submit myself completely to God, but I find **I can't even do that lest He show me.**

The promise is, **"Submit to God, resist the devil, and he will flee from you!"** (James 4:7 NKJV).

Our inner Holy Spirit guides us into all truth. As we learn of God's incredible love for each of us, then the more we love God back. The more we love God back, the more you'll find you're loving *yourself* more little by little!

In our most difficult days of fasting, we can do it! Submit to God, resist the devil, and he will flee from you! And don't entice your own fleshly desires that will drag you away!

Let God. Just let God.

Prayer: *Father, in the holy name of Jesus, I praise and thank You over and over again because this* New Godly Eating Lifestyle© *makes me more grateful to be alive every day! I'm beginning to see the hope of my future and the good plans You have for me.*

I pray and fast today for:

____

____

____

Remind me to submit, resist and win! Please, Lord, any time that I am tempted, please show me the way of escape! As I embrace The A.N.G.E.L. Plan: A New Godly Eating Lifestyle©, *keep me safe from all satan's attacks, no matter where they come from. In the name of Jesus, amen.*

42

Ask, and it will be given to you;
seek, and you will find;
knock, and it will be opened to you.
(Matthew 7:7 NKJV)

One of the most frustrating things about "dieting" is to do good all day long, all week long, or even all month long, and the scale doesn't even budge an ounce! **Throw the scales away!** The scales can blind you to what is really going on in your body overall, not just for a moment or for a day. The scales may also encourage body dysmorphic disorder. **Again, throw away your scales! Feel your body in your looser clothes!**

The true beauty of *The A.N.G.E.L. Plan©* is that **incorporating the three basic elements (lots of prayer + lots of water + 7/17 intermittent fasting) can change your entire way of thinking, your entire way of eating, and your entire life!**

In Matthew 7:7, Jesus promised that I can **(1) ask and it will be given, (2) seek and I shall find, and (3) knock and it shall be opened to me.**

We can barely comprehend its meaning—God may do it for someone else, but **do we believe God will do it for us? He promises that He will. Ask. Seek. Knock.**

*Prayer: Holy Lord, in the name of Jesus, I bring my **thanksgiving and praise to You today** because of Your incredible love, mercy, and grace, and mostly because I love and adore You, oh Lord! **May You receive my thanksgiving and my praise throughout all eternity!***

I pray and fast today for:

____

____

____

Please help me to depend entirely on You, Father, in the power of the Holy Spirit, *so that I might know You and love You more and better!*

Please help me to depend on the feel of my clothes and body to count my progress, instead of me paying homage to the scales.

We love, praise, thank and worship You, in the name of Jesus, amen and amen.

43

Everyone who thirsts,
Come to the waters;
And you who have no money,
Come, buy and eat.
Yes, come, buy wine and milk
Without money and without price.
Why do you spend money
for what is not bread,
And your wages for
what does not satisfy?
Listen carefully to Me,
and eat what is good,
And let your soul delight
itself in abundance.
Incline your ear, and come to Me.
Hear, and your soul shall live....
(Isaiah 55:1 NKJV)

As a Christian, **you owe it to yourself to have all of the bene-fits** of *The A.N.G.E.L. Plan©*!

If you feel you've tried and couldn't make it, **LOOK AGAIN!** Go back over Chapter 11, *The A.N.G.E.L. Plan: A New Godly Eating Lifestyle©* of this book and see what you've been forgetting or not fully doing daily. I have had to do this at various times since embracing *A New Godly Eating Lifestyle©*. Go back and check yourself as often as you need—**I suggest every morning for the first ten days.**

The intense sense of full freedom from food addiction is a fleshly joy like none I've ever known! I wish I could fully express that freedom to you, but it is something you can and will find for yourself in *The A.N.G.E.L. Plan©*.

*Prayer: Jehovah God, our provider, our redeemer, our greatest love, our Father, our Savior, our Messiah, and our inner Holy Ghost, **I thank You and praise You** for **Who You are** and all that You've done for me and continue to do for me moment by moment, in Your perfect timing.*

I pray and fast today for:

____

____

____

Help me, Father, to fully embrace A New Godly Eating Lifestyle©, *and let it become **a part of my everyday existence.** May* The A.N.G.E.L. Plan© *feel as natural to me as breathing! In the name of Jesus, amen.*

44

So shall My word be
that goes forth from My mouth;
It shall not return to Me void,
But it shall accomplish what I please,
And it shall prosper in the thing
for which I sent it.
For you shall go out with joy,
And be led out with peace;
The mountains and the hills
break forth into singing before you,
And all the trees of the field
shall clap their hands.
(Isaiah 55:11–12 NKJV)

God's Words (whether the written Holy Bible or His *rhema* Word in our spirit) are just the way it is. **God doesn't change, nor does He go back on His Word.** When things are happening in the spirit and finally manifesting in the natural, then shall we know

- that God is working,
- that God is good all the time,
- that God's timing is perfect,
- that every action God takes or prayer that He answers depends on our faith in His Word, and
- that God's Word will not return to Him void of the promises that He has made.

The second part of our verse for the day talks about the most supreme of topics: **JOY and PEACE! God directs us to go out with JOY! If so, we will be led out in PEACE.** Going about our day in JOY and PEACE causes positive actions in the natural world—the mountains and hills break forth with singing! All the trees of the field shall clap their hands! (Isaiah 55:12–12).

SEEK YOUR JOY!

There is a place that we can reach when we can have **internal** and **eternal** JOY, regardless of the circumstances we are in or that surround us—threats in the future in our finances or gaining a pound or two.

The scales or our weight should never determine our joy!

We cannot be fully grateful to God if we have not reached a place of internal JOY in our lives. We want to live **knowing** that God's got our back, that we are not on a diet, but we know and are still learning that *The A.N.G.E.L. Plan©* works, and we can trust ourselves to its processes and God's promises.

Prayer: Father, in the name of Jesus, I THANK YOU and PRAISE YOU for Your many, many answers to my prayers, and for the prayers that You did not answer because You love me and want Your best for me.

I pray and fast today for:

____

____

____

Help me, Lord, to seek and find my JOY and PEACE in YOU!
May I never expect any person, place, or thing to be the source of my JOY!

I thank you, Lord, that Your Word and Your promises in it will never return to You void. Thank You that Your Word and promises accomplish Your intention all along—that I should know goodness and mercy all the days of my life as I dwell in Your presence forever. Amen.

45

Behold, I am with you and
will keep you wherever you go....
For I will not leave you until I have
done what I have spoken to you.
(Genesis 28:15 NKJV)

Our Father taught us, as early as Genesis 28, that He is with us wherever we go. The Bible says in many places, **"Fear not, for I am with you."** That is the only reason that God tells us not to fear is **because He is with us wherever we go.**

God also promises us that He will not leave us until He has done what He has spoken to us. That promise means different things to different people in different circumstances.

Perhaps, you too feel that God has spoken to you, and you can also rest in His promises that He will not stop working on your behalf until He has done as He promised.

Be still. Know that He is God. Listen for His voice and learn to wait patiently to hear Him. You'll soon be tuning in sooner than you think.

Learn to be led by His "still, small voice" in your inner Spirit, and always welcome Him into your presence and prayer time with thanksgiving and praise!

*Prayer: Heavenly Father, in Jesus's holy and precious name, I give You thanks and praise for all that You have done, **and are doing** in, in my life! I am learning to be content and even happy during either my fasting times or "feasting" times, and I thank You that I'm learning to desire and to eat healthy foods instead of junk.*

Keep me, oh, Lord, so that I may today resist all the fiery darts of the enemy with Your Word, the sword of the Spirit, the breastplate of righteousness, and the helmet of salvation. May I walk adorned with the belt of truth and my feet going forth with the gospel of peace.

I pray and fast today for:

____

____

____

In the name of Jesus, amen.

46

So kill (deaden, deprive of power)
the evil desire lurking in your members
*[those animal impulses and all that is
earthly in you that is employed in sin]:*
***sexual vice, impurity, sensual
appetites, unholy desires, and all
greed and covetousness,
for that is idolatry***
*(the deifying of self and other
created things instead of God).*
(Colossians 3:5 AMPC)

What is your favorite thing to do? What is your favorite thing to wear? What is your favorite thing to say? What is your favorite thing to eat?

Check each of your answers and compare them to the importance of God in your own life. You and only you know whether or not your desires are evil and employed in sin, or whether they are thoughts and desires to please God in Jesus Christ.

God's first commandment given to Moses is, **"Thou shalt have no other gods before me"** (Exodus 20:3 KJV).

Jesus told His disciples that the first and greatest commandment was,

**Thou shalt love the Lord thy God with all thy heart,
and with all thy soul, and
with all thy mind.
This is the first and great commandment.**
(Matthew 22:37–38 KJV)

It is only through renewing our minds with the Word of God that we are transformed into that new creation we are promised. Dead to sin and alive in Jesus Christ eternally!

As we make God our first priority in life, all other priorities seem to just fall into place. It's a God deal in God's perfect timing.

Prayer: Father, Lord Jesus, Holy Spirit thank You again and again for all the blessings I know and am aware of when I keep You absolutely first in my life. Help me to keep my eyes, my heart and soul completely focused on Your will before anything or anyone else.

Thank You for The A.N.G.E.L. Plan© and all the benefits I've felt and seen since I changed my eating lifestyle and opted for the truths in Your Word. Keep me from temptation Lord and let me always see the way out that You have promised to show me.

I pray and fast today for:

____

____

____

Father, I love, thank, and praise You in Jesus's most holy name, amen!

47

*Let us hold fast
the confession of our Hope
without wavering,
for He Who promised IS Faithful!*
(Hebrews 10:23 NKJV)

Most of us believe by now that God is assisting and directing our new eating lifestyle as we endeavor to become **all** God wants us to be. Many of us hear from the Lord through His *rhema* word promises or written promises in His Word, and this scripture is especially encouraging and exciting! **God, Who promised, is faithful!**

No matter how we may become discouraged—whether with our personal attempts to defeat the dance with diets or to weather an attack from the enemy out of absolutely nowhere! Because things sometimes do just happen out of nowhere, we must always go to God first. We can be hit like a hurricane with undeserved, uncalled for, totally irrational attacks from the enemy, who will try with all his might to steer us away from *The A.N.G.E.L. Plan*© and our *New Godly Eating Lifestyle*©. satan hates our progress because he does not want us to have victory over any of our spiritually or physically destructive eating patterns!

As you begin to relax now, sit back, contemplate, and enjoy the effects of *A New Godly Eating Lifestyle*©, including renewed vitality, extra energy, and **freedom** from enslavement to eating. If you've come this far, the positive effects of *The A.N.G.E.L. Plan*© are happening for you now! As the writer of Hebrews tells us today and every day, **"Let us hold fast the confession of our Hope without wavering, for He Who promised is faithful!"** (Hebrews 10:23 NKJV).

During dark times, we must turn **first to God instead of to food**. Never ever turn to food to salve dark feelings or on seemingly dark days. Reach up and out to God and you will be pleasing Him and will receive His help.

*Prayer: Our Father in heaven, holy is Your name, Your kingdom come, Your will be done on earth as it is in heaven. Please give us this day our **daily bread** and forgive us our sins **as we forgive those who sin against us**. And lead us not into temptation, Lord, but **please deliver us from evil**. For thine is the kingdom, the power, and the glory now and forever. Amen!*

I pray and fast today for:

____

____

____

Father, I love, thank, and praise You in the most holy name of Jesus, amen!

48

Why are you cast down, O my soul?
And why are you in turmoil within me?
Hope in God
for I shall again praise Him,
my Salvation and my God.
(*Psalms 42:11 ESV*)

Some days, I just wake up in a funk. Nothing's really wrong, or things may be really wrong, yet some days, I can still wake up in a funk either way. Maybe you can relate.

I may just not be ready for prayer that morning—for the first few minutes at least. Yet the depths of my soul reach out to greet Jesus first thing because I have learned that my soul's satisfaction is my only really important need in my life. That is the peace and the joy I find in my morning "walks in the garden" with Him. Or on my morning trips to the bathroom with Him… Just get away with Him for a few moments or a few hours if I can.

Those days, as all days, I have to remind myself to approach the Father with THANKSGIVING and PRAISE! He tells us to enter His courts with them!

And then, following Jesus's directive in the Sermon on the Mount, I have to ask the Lord to search me and my heart and forgive me of my sins and weaknesses, *in accordance with* the way I am willing to forgive all others. I have to look back over who I might have hurt recently and seek forgiveness from God and from them.

Then I need to just be still and listen… Listen to the quiet, listen to praise music or teachings, all the while listening for the still small voice of God.

As I do that faithfully each day, the enemy starts off defeated! I can go forward and seek the "daily bread" that I need; and I give my day, my will, thoughts, attitudes, expressions, reactions, and choices under captivity to the obedience of Christ (2 Corinthians 10:4–5 KJV).

This way, food has no say in how I choose to conduct my day, regardless of how I "feel" when I wake up. Feelings lie and they are fleeting… **I must stand on what I've learned so far and depend on God to deliver me out of all temptation.**

Prayer: Heavenly Father, in the awesome and mighty name of Jesus, I come before You with PRAISE and THANKSGIVING for what You have already done and are already doing, and thank You that You have helped me this far in The A.N.G.E.L. Plan©!

I pray and fast today for:

____

____

____

Once again, I offer You PRAISE and THANKSGIVING and ask that You please strengthen me today to resist all the fiery darts and temptations of the enemy. In the name of Jesus, amen and amen.

49

*Now the Lord is the Spirit, and
where the Spirit of the Lord is,
there is liberty.*
(2 Corinthians 3:17 NKJV)

When we step into the spiritual realm for praise, thanksgiving, and prayer, we address our thoughts and prayers and conversation with the one and only Lord of hosts!

The Holy Spirit or Holy Ghost, and Christ, the Son, and the Heavenly Father are all spirits. **What a fantastic promise to us that when we seek out and follow the Spirit of the Lord, there is indeed LIBERTY—true freedom and "emancipation from bondage"!**

YOU CAN BE EMANCIPATED FROM SLAVERY TO FOOD AND THE BONDAGE AND MENTAL HELL THAT COMES WITH THAT ENSLAVEMENT!

First, above all things, we must **SEEK THE LORD—HIS GLORY AND POWER AND MAJESTY AND BEAUTY AND HIS AWESOME LOVE FOR "ME"!** For where the Spirit of the Lord is, there is freedom!

Prayer: Heavenly Father, in the precious name of Jesus, I just want to love You and praise You and thank You for all my prayers answered in Your due time. Help me not to be impatient, but to trust that You will give me just what I need at just Your appointed time.

I pray and fast today for:

____

____

____

May I rest in Your divine presence *regardless of what I'm doing throughout this day and night, and keep me close to Your heart, oh God! In the name of Jesus! Amen.*

50

No temptation has overtaken you
except such as is common to man;
but God is faithful,
Who will not allow you to be tempted
beyond what you are able,
but with the temptation will also make
the way of escape,
that you may be able to bear it.
(1 Corinthians 10:13 NKJV)

While this is a most comforting scripture, it is one of the hardest to face. It may seem I'm trying, praying, fasting to break a "bad habit" as yet to no avail. I can look at this scripture over and over, while continuing in the Bad Habit. I can know God has made a way of escape, yet sometimes I may flat refuse to actually use that escape route!

We can consciously or unconsciously know that we are willingly going down a path that leads to our biggest temptations, and if we check our true motive, we are actually trying to set ourselves up. For a failure? I hope not.

Failure is NOT necessary!

When we feel our strong will rise up against the truths that we know, and we reject one of God's escape routes, we immediately feel shame and a surge of desire to hide from God, just as Adam and Eve did.

Today, I am depending on God's mercy and grace and eternal patience with me to help me to break this Bad Habit and to forgive me for times when I've given in.

Prayer: Dear Father, today I come to You to ask for You to forgive my known and unknown sin, my willful sin, in continuing to engage in this unhealthy habit.

I am willing to give this bad habit up to You, Lord. Please help me.

Help my unbelief and let my mouth declare that I am walking and living in freedom from bondage as You lead me through this "valley of the shadow of death."

I pray and fast today for:

____

____

____

Father, I love, thank, and praise You in the most holy name of Jesus, amen!

51

When tempted, no one should say,
"God is tempting me."
For God cannot be tempted by evil,
nor does He tempt anyone;
but each person is tempted
when they are dragged away
by their own evil desire and enticed.
(James 1:13–14 NIV)

Wow! There is probably no greater truth than verse 14 above regarding our sins, temptations, and overeating. We usually just "set ourselves up" by accidentally driving by Braum's or Freddy's or old Macky D's, and we just happen to turn in there, unplanned and unexpectedly. We can actually talk about a certain food so much that we totally override every defense we have about that particular food. **Don't "romance" food!**

God, however, will never ever tempt us! It is satan and his little minions that are tempting and tickling our flesh to overindulge, to not eat at all, or to eat ourselves literally beyond recognition!

For overeaters, have you noticed that when your weight is "down" and you feel good, your face is smaller and your smile is far more attractive as well? God's achievements in you make satan as angry as hell!

satan wants to ruin your smile and your beautiful facial features that God designed specifically for you! satan wants to distort you by adding pounds to distort your features, squint your eyes, add extra chins, make it hard to move around, et cetera, and to allow you no way to enjoy life! He certainly wants to rob you of your joy of the Lord. If satan can rob you of your joy, he can rob you of your strength. "The joy of the Lord is my strength," the old hymn says.

Prayer: Father God, I ask for Your anointing today to accomplish my fasting and healthy eating. I find it ever so hard—sometimes too hard—to try my daily fasting or even my feasting without You, oh, Lord.

Father, we ask that as we follow The A.N.G.E.L. Plan© *that You restore to us the beauty that You designed in each of us as we get healthier and have more vitality and, most importantly, to grow in our love for and knowledge of You!*

I pray and fast today for:

____

____

____

In the name of Jesus, amen and amen!

52

Fear not, for I am with you;
Be not dismayed, for I am your God.
I will strengthen you,
Yes, I will help you,
I will uphold you
With my righteous right hand.
(Isaiah 41:10 NKJV)

What is the great answer to the world's problems? Jesus said the greatest commandments are these: **"You shall love the Lord your God with all your heart, soul mind and strength. And a second is like it, you shall love your neighbor as yourself"** (Matthew 22:37–38). **Imagine how great the world would be!**

Each morning, as you approach your time of prayer and meditation and spending your own special time with God, search your heart and mind and emotions and see if there is anyone, any person or entity, whom you are mad at or hold some anger or unforgiveness. **Resolve your unforgiveness, pray for anyone who has hurt you, and do not talk negatively about them.**

When we can do these things in the morning, we are able to approach God more humbly and to give him PRAISE and THANKSGIVING for all of the blessings in our lives! Just start with counting your blessings—your salvation, for God's people, animals, places, seen and unseen things!

Count your blessings and *reach in and find your joy of the Lord*! You'll find it much easier to commit yourself to your *A.N.G.E.L. Plan©* when you've prepared yourself in this way.

Prayer: Father, thank You for revealing Your Godly eating life-style—a way to healthy weight without having to "diet" ever again! As I grow more day by day in You, I thank You for my freedom from the

bondage and enslavement to food, thoughts of food, planning food, and impulsively making food choices!
I pray and fast today for:

____

____

____

In the name of Jesus, amen!

53

I waited patiently for the Lord,
And He inclined to me, and
Heard my cry.
He also brought me out of
A horrible pit,
Out of the miry clay, and
Set my feet upon a Rock, and
Established my steps.
(Psalm 40:1–2 NKJV)

Just how are we tempted? Seeing the bad habit practiced in front of us; advertisements; emails and other spam; hanging with friends who practice the bad habit themselves.

The Bible shows that we can be led astray in two general ways: satan puts temptations in our way either through tempting us to excess foods; or we are enticed and led astray by our own fleshly desires.

In either case, God promises that He will always provide a way out of the temptation without having to resort to overeating, binging, or purging.

Prayer: Precious Father, I THANK AND PRAISE YOU for The A.N.G.E.L. Plan©, and I ask Your anointing on me to break that bad habit once and for all, holy Lord.

Make me aware when I am being enticed by my fleshly desires so I cannot be led astray by satan or my own mental processes.

I pray and fast today for:

____

____

____

*In the precious name of **Jesus, which is mightier than any other name,** amen!*

54

*My brethren, count it all JOY
When you fall into various trials,
Knowing that the testing of your
Faith produces patience.*
(James 1:2–3 NKJV)

This is a very comforting scripture once we realize that GOD's JOY is one of the greatest "gifts" we can seek from our Father in heaven. When we truly have God's joy in our spirit, mind, and mouth, then we are comforted in knowing that when we pass the trials and the tests of our faith, we will have also learned a whole lot about the fruit of patience, one of the fruits of the Spirit.

God NEVER, EVER tempts us, and He promises that He will always provide a way out of the temptation if we lean into and look to Him for the right path. God said He will guide us with His eye, and if we're filled with the Holy Spirit, He definitely does guide us. Learn to "lean into" Him for your greatest joy and comfort.

However, we must be very, very careful to "try the spirits to see if they are of God," to make certain that we are not just being led astray.

*Prayer: Dear Lord, in the precious name of Jesus, I want to pause—to actually **stop and thank You and praise You** for all the many, many blessings in my life—those blessings that fall on me daily that I often take for granted, and my many answered (and unanswered) prayers that You and I discuss daily.*

I thank You and praise You that You have already provided for my basic needs and that my prayers, according to Your will, are now coming into fruition.

I pray and fast today for:

____

____

____

Father, thank You so much for The A.N.G.E.L. Plan©, *and I pray that You help me during my fasting and feasting times today. In the holy and majestic name of Jesus, amen and amen!*

55

In **Matthew 6 of the Sermon on the Mount,**
Jesus taught the people in this order to:
Give
Pray
Forgive
Fast

Jesus immediately taught us to pray and fast after He taught giving and then forgiving, as a natural part of our joyful everyday life! It's not too hard for us or Jesus would not have taught us to do it!

YOU can give, pray, forgive, AND fast! God will bless you in doing so, and He will give you the strength to find ways of escape and ways out of temptation.

Prayer: Father, in the mighty name of Jesus, I love and thank and praise You for all my many, many blessings and so many answered prayers!

Help me, Lord, to forgive immediately those who have hurt or offended me and to make things right as soon as possible. Give to me that I might bless others to meet their needs and to spread Your Word around the world.

Help me to pray without ceasing, that I might intercede for the lost and the lonely, the sick, and the lame, both mentally and spiritually.

Help me to commit to the fast that You would have me do today and help me, Lord, to beware of the enemy in his many different guises and blindfolds!

I pray and fast today for:

____

____

____

Praising You, Father, praising the name of Jesus, and praise the endless power of the Holy Spirit of the Trinity—God, Christ, and the Holy Ghost!

56

**But when you fast,
anoint your head
and wash your face,
that your fasting may not
be seen by others
but by your Father who is in secret.
And your Father who sees in secret will reward you.**
(Matthew 6:17–18 ESV)

Jesus, the Word, and God the Father told us how our fasting should be done. It's really very simple—wash your face, anoint your head (and groom yourself) so that you don't appear to be fasting.

By the time you've reached this fifty-sixth devotion, you have experienced progress in your body, you've certainly grown in the Spirit, and you've heard many compliments, you even believe God is pleased with you! Thus, you may be tempted to take credit for your own progress, your own weight loss, your own physical health.

REMEMBER, ALL OF OUR PROGRESS IS FOR THE *GLORY OF GOD*!

Start your day off on point with your morning prayer and devotions, being watchful and prayerful as you consider your fasting and feasting for the day.

Prayer: Father, in the name of Jesus, please help me to keep my daily priorities straight. Remind me to thank and praise You every time I lift my thoughts toward You and open my eyes to Your beauty all around me!

I pray and fast today for:

____

____

____

Father, please accomplish in me today whatever Your heart wills that I do, and I thank You for a wonderful day ahead! In the holy and mighty name of Jesus, amen!

57

Don't worry about anything;
instead, pray about everything.
Tell God what you need,
and thank Him for all He has done.
(Philippians 4:6 NLT)

Some days seem to magnetically draw the worst to us *and* bring out the worst in us! Some days challenge our character and courage each step of the way.

It's impossible to walk in faith and fear at the same time. Faith dispels fear just as light dispels darkness.

God never tells us to hurry to finish our prayers. No, He invites us into lengthy conversations and times of fellowship with Him! We are the ones who end prayer first, and **often we fail to take the time to listen for God's replies**, *rhema* words and instructions.

When those days come on us suddenly or it's a planned adventure that turns sour, your hope is always in Jesus the Christ. He is the all-powerful God Who has chosen your path for you. **Trust Him!**

Prayer: Father, in the name of Jesus, please draw me into closer fellowship with You. Help me to tune into the voice of the Holy Spirit as easily as possible because I long to have more of You!

I pray and fast today for:

____
____
____

In the holy and glorious name of Jesus, amen.

58

*For your obedience has
become known to all.
Therefore I am glad on your behalf;
but I want you to be wise in what is good,
and simple concerning evil.
And the God of peace will crush
satan under your feet shortly.
The grace of
our Lord Jesus Christ
be with you.
Amen.*
(Romans 16:19-20 NKJV)

Every day that we intentionally embrace *The A.N.G.E.L. Plan*©, it becomes easier and easier to accomplish until the Plan becomes automatic. Fasting becomes easier and easier, and you find that your ability to live *The A.N.G.E.L. Plan*© grows daily.

When you reach that place in your *New Godly Eating Lifestyle*© where you find daily 7/17 fasting automatic, and you may look forward to your feast days—for me Sunday and a weekday—then you have indeed reached a milestone in *your New Godly Eating Lifestyle*©.

Does this mean that you quit?

No! You have a brand, new lifestyle that will keep you out of eating disorderly hell and which SETS YOU FREE FROM THE BONDAGE OF FOOD!

You may want to cut back a day of fasting when you reach your goal weight. God will show you how to eat daily to maintain your food freedom!

Prayer: Father, I thank You and praise You that Your love and Your Holy Spirit have enabled me to adapt to A New Godly Eating

Lifestyle©. *Thank You for the miraculous changes in my health and in my physical body, oh, Lord!*

Give me someone to share A New Godly Eating Lifestyle© **with,** *and may I use Your wisdom and love and tact to speak what I should speak.* **Help me not to be pushy or condemning,** *but to speak of Your glory and Your majesty and Your infinite grace and mercy in* The A.N.G.E.L. Plan©.

I pray and fast today for:

____

____

____

I love You and thank You for the blessings and answers that You have already sent my way, in Jesus's mighty name, amen!

59

For the word of God is
living and powerful,
and sharper than any
two-edged sword,
piercing even to the
division of soul and spirit,
and of joints and marrow,
and is a discerner of the
thoughts and
intents of the heart.
(Hebrews 4:12 NKJV)

What we say about ourselves becomes our reality. Spoken words have creative power—that is how the world was created! **When we speak positive words about ourselves to ourselves and to others, we change the flow of creative power from negative to positive.**

What is also important is to not allow others to say negative words to you or over you! **We must set them straight right away in a peaceful tone.** I have learned that the more we respect ourselves, the more others will respect us too.

When you start your day, say some positive things about yourself. Look straight into your mirror and admire yourself with a beautiful eye. Develop some affirmations to add to your morning routine.

In chapter 14, **I have included sixty of my own affirmations that I've gathered throughout the years which you may find helpful, and you can write your own specific affirmations also. Reading them out loud in *your* voice often keeps them fresh in your mind and will change your way of thinking about yourself!**

They will help you know who *you* are *in Christ*!

Put God's Words in your mouth and praise and gratitude into your speech, and you will have started a very good day!

Prayer: Father, in the powerful and mighty name of Jesus, I thank You and praise You and love You all the more day by day! I love that You love me more than I can possibly imagine!

I thank You that Your Word is creative and powerful, and I pray that You put Your Words in my mind and mouth that I may follow my Godly Eating Lifestyle© today and every day.

I pray and fast today for:

____

____

____

In Jesus's holy name, amen and amen!

60

*Put on the whole armor of God,
that you may be able to stand against
the wiles of the devil....
Stand therefore, having girded
your waist with truth,
having put on the breastplate
of righteousness, and
having shod your feet with the
preparation of the Gospel of peace;
above all, taking the shield of faith...
And take the helmet of salvation, and
the sword of the Spirit,
which is the word of God;*
**Praying always with all prayer and
supplication in the Spirit,
being watchful to this end with all
perseverance and supplication
for all the saints—.**
(Ephesians 6:11, 14–15, 17–18 NKJV)

We truly are at war with evil and demonic powers in high places and in our eating habits, smoking habits, drinking habits, spending habits, *ad infinitum.*

I love my morning time with God, where I can praise, worship, and give thanks for His eternal goodness and for His immeasurable love just for me and for you too! I can listen to teaching or read a good spiritual book. If I'm in ministry, I can extend my morning time to work on those things for which He has called me to do. My time with Him and my ministry are not the same thing. We must take time for both.

Morning devotion prepares me for my day, especially if I take the time to **"Put on the whole armor of God that [I] may be able**

to stand against the wiles of the devil" (Ephesians 6:11). When I've awakened early to spend as much time as possible with the Lord, my day goes much more peacefully and profitably than if I had not.

I cannot overemphasize the importance of morning devotions in *The A.N.G.E.L. Plan—A New Godly Eating Lifestyle©*.

> ***Therefore take up the whole armor of God,***
> ***that you may be able to withstand***
> ***in the evil day, and***
> ***having done all, to stand.***
> *(Ephesians 6:14 NKJV)*

Prayer: Father, in the precious name of Jesus, I thank You and praise You and love You for giving me The A.N.G.E.L. Plan—New Godly Eating Lifestyle©. *I thank You that I've made it through this book of devotions and that I have immersed myself and fully committed myself to* The A.N.G.E.L. Plan©.

I pray and fast today for:

____

____

____

Father, Lord Jesus, and precious Holy Spirit Who give me self-control, thank You that I don't have to live on a diet rollercoaster anymore! In the most holy name of Jesus, amen and amen.

14

Prayers of Blessings

HOW JESUS
TAUGHT US TO PRAY

In the beginning of the New Testament, Matthew 6:9–13 (NKJV), **Jesus said,**

In this manner, therefore, Pray:
"Our Father in Heaven,
Hallowed be Your name.
Your Kingdom come.
Your will be done on earth
as it is in Heaven.
Give us this day our daily bread.
And forgive us our debts,
as we forgive our debtors.
And lead us not into temptation
but deliver us from the evil one.
For Yours is the kingdom
and the
power and the glory forever!"
Amen.

PRAYER WHEN TEMPTED

My dear Father, Jehovah Jirah! Abba, Father—my Savior and Comforter and my God! Thank You that you are more than willing to come immediately to my aid in times of temptation or physical hunger during my fasting periods, and I pray, sweet Holy Spirit, rise up in me and keep me from overeating or thinking of junk food during my times of feasting!

Let my New Godly Eating Lifestyle© *become second nature to me until it becomes my true nature!*

I love You and praise You and glorify You for Who You are, my God, and I thank You that You alone are more than enough to give me the strength to do this today! In the glorious name of Jesus, amen and amen!

> But when you fast, anoint your head and wash your face, that your fasting may not be seen by others but by your Father who is in secret. And your Father who sees in secret will reward you. (Matthew 6:17–18 ESV)

PRAYER TO BE LED BY THE HOLY SPIRIT

Holy Father, in the mighty and precious name of Jesus, I am utterly helpless in my own strength to deal with this thorn in my flesh of addiction to food and cravings that seem utterly overwhelming. May Your Holy Spirit lead me out of temptation and lead the way to my victory over food enslavement, so that food no longer rules my thoughts, mind, will, emotions, or actions in eating; but that I see it as nothing other than fuel to my body.

Jesus, You are the strength of my spirit, soul, and mind! In Your strength, I can follow The A.N.G.E.L. Plan©! Amen and amen.

DAILY PRAYER AND MEDITATION

"I CAN DO ALL THINGS THROUGH CHRIST WHO STRENGTHENS ME!" (Philippians 4:13 NKJV).

PRAYER FOR HUMILITY

*Father, as I see so many of Your children around me who are obviously in a battle with food and their weight, give me a heart of empathy for them and may I never criticize another heavy person again because **"but for the grace of God go I!"** May I gladly share* A New Godly Eating Lifestyle© *with anyone who needs or wants to know.* **In the holy name of Jesus,** *amen!*

PRAYER TO STAND AGAINST THE ENEMY

Our awesome Maker, MY Creator, and the Creator of all things, thank You that no weapon—even weapons of my own devise—formed against me shall prosper or enjoy any success!

Thank You that You allow no temptation beyond what I am able to stand, and that YOU WILL ALWAYS provide a way out!

Help those who have chosen The A.N.G.E.L. Plan©, *as we walk the path toward healthy living, feeling, and looking the best we can, but only for Your glory, honor, and praise. In the holy name of Jesus, amen.*

PRAYER TO LOVE GOD BACK!

*Holy God and Heavenly Papa, thank You that **You are both** to me! Your Holiness and Grace and Love and Mercy bring me to my knees, yet **I know that as my Papa, I can rest my head in Your lap, dear Lord.***

I thank You that You know what I need - and that Your provisions are already on the way <u>before</u> I even know I need them! Thank You that TODAY miracles will happen to me as I thank and praise my way through my day, loving You back with all my heart and soul and mind! In the name of Jesus, Amen!

PRAYER FOR PATIENCE

*Father, as we think about growing in the fruit of the Spirit of patience, help us to surrender to the Holy Spirit, **letting "self" go.** Please remind me, Lord, that trials will always test our faith, and **the testing*** *of our faith in You produces patience and many other fruit of Your Spirit!* I thank You that patience is having its perfect work in me, that I may be complete, lacking nothing! In the name of Jesus, amen!

PRAYER TO GUARD YOUR MIND

Holy Father, in the precious, glorious, and mighty name of Jesus, **forgive me of my sins and negativity and doubt. Please forgive me as I forgive others, my Lord, and help me to forgive them through You, Jesus, that I might receive Your forgiveness and find joy and peace.**

Help me, please, Lord, to bring my mind, thoughts, emotions, words, expressions, actions, reactions, motives, and my very will completely captive to the obedience of Christ moment by moment! Help me… Change me as only You can! *In the name of Jesus, amen.*

PRAYER OF THANKSGIVING

Abba Father, Lord God, deep down, **I know in my heart what You have genuinely done for me, and continue to do for me, those things I cannot do for myself.** *As I learn to walk in* **the self-discipline of the Holy Spirit,** *help me to make good choices that are healthy and satisfying to me.*

Thank you that I am not deprived of any food, and **I have the newfound freedom to fast and to eat as YOU will, Lord, under the discipline of the Holy Spirit, which I already have!** *In the holy and miraculous name of Jesus, amen and amen!*

NOW MAKE A GRATITUDE LIST

PRAYER ABOUT JEALOUSY

Father, in the holy and precious name of Jesus, hear my cry, oh, Lord! Please just help me. Help me in the way You know I need. **Please reveal to me the reasons why I choose to turn to food instead of to YOU, Lord God.**

*I ask that **You take away jealousy in every form** within me and help me please to find REST in YOU in my heart and soul, in my mind, my will, my thoughts and my emotions. I ask the same for my spouse, Lord!*

***I thank You that You have already prepared answers to my prayers and they're on the way!** I give all the credit to You, my Lord and my Savior, and please help me each step of the way! Hallelujah! And Amen!*

PRAYER TO SUBMIT OUR SOUL TO GOD

Father, in Jesus's precious name, I submit my mind, thoughts, will, emotions, words, and expressions into captivity to the obedience of Christ.

Please help me because I know deep down in my inner core that I cannot bear this journey of life or A New Godly Eating Lifestyle© without Your help every step of the way. I pray, dear Father, that I will not give in to temptation for I know that "my Spirit is willing, but my body is weak." Thank You for all that You are! In the name of Jesus, amen.

PRAYER FOR LOVE, LIFE, AND LIVING WATER

*Dear Father, Lord Jesus, Holy Ghost, enrapture me in Your love and Your rest and take away the physical desires for excess food—food beyond my need, and help me, Lord—**HELP ME, PLEASE—to be satisfied in You** rather than food or drink.*

***Jesus, YOU are the Bread of Life and the Living Water**, and I thank YOU over and over and over for giving me freedom from enslavement to worry, anxiety, stress, guilt, jealousy, gluttony, and food!*

Enable and remind me, Lord, please, to complete my daily water intake of four to six 16-oz glasses or bottles of water today.

PRAYER FOR PEACE

*Father, I pray for Your **peace** in my life, in my spouse, my children and their children, and for **peace** in my home as only YOU can give. I will be a peacemaker. In Your precious and most holy name! Amen and amen.*

PRAYER TO LIVE IN GOD'S PERFECT TIMING

Father, as I go through this wonderful day, remind me often of the beauty that surrounds me, the smiles and the laughter, the inherent goodness of a human being, and the true wonders of your world. Selah.

You flung the stars into space and made the sun to warm your people and give them light! You did it all in an orderly fashion and in Your perfect timing!

You and Your perfect timing control all Your inhabitants of the universe, oh, God!

I thank You, Almighty Father, that You have put my life in Your perfect timing, and that You are never late (even if You show Yourself after death, as was the case with Lazarus)!

May I trust today and every day that my entire life is in Your perfect timing, that I may relax and do the next right thing, rather than trying to tackle all my problems at once.

***As I delight myself in Your ways (and I certainly do), I thank You, Father, that You will make my crooked paths straight and lead me beside green pastures and still waters. Lord, please grant all of my heart's greatest desires which I can handle while keeping You first of all…all in* Your perfect timing!**

I pray and I thank and I praise you, Father, in the holy, majestic, and precious name of Jesus! Amen and amen.

15

Affirmations

The following are sixty affirmations that I personally use. You can try them or just write your own. Either way, you will **immediately** feel better!

WHO AM I?
WHO AM I *IN CHRIST*?

1. "I CAN DO ALL THINGS THROUGH CHRIST WHO STRENGTHENS ME!"
2. I bring my MIND, WILL, THOUGHTS, EMOTIONS, ACTIONS, REACTIONS, EXPRESSIONS, AND ALL MY WORDS into CAPTIVITY TO THE OBEDIENCE OF CHRIST daily!
3. I have the mind of Christ, who has all knowledge, all wisdom, all power and faithfulness! (I can find lost things when I ask Christ's help to locate them.)
4. My memory improves daily!
5. I am miraculously and wonderfully saved by His matchless love, His forgiveness, His mercy, and His eternal grace!
6. MIRACLES SHOW UP REGULARLY IN MY LIFE, AND ANOTHER IS COMING TODAY!
7. I am becoming MORE AND MORE AWARE OF MY ANGELS and their ministry to me. I will learn more about them.

8. I am blessed!

9. I am talented in areas I've never even explored!

10. I am LOSING WEIGHT DAILY until I become the weight that God would have me!

11. I am a GREAT WIFE!

12. I am faithful.

13. I am loyal.

14. I am funny.

15. I love to laugh!

16. I do NOT feel sorry for myself for any reason!

17. I AM A CHILD OF THE MOST HIGH GOD, AN HEIR TO SALVATION AND TO ALL GOOD THINGS HERE ON EARTH AND IN HEAVEN FOR ETER-NITY!

18. I am beautiful inside and out!

19. I am learning to love myself more each day, and therefore, I can more fully love God and others.

20. I have HOPE for a great future!

21. Yay, though I walk through the valley of the shadow of death, I will fear no evil, for Thy rod and Thy staff shall comfort me, deliver me, and keep the predators away all the days of my life, and I will dwell in the House of the Lord forever!

22. He makes me LIE DOWN in green pastures when I am tired and hungry.

23. He prepares a table before me in the presence of my ene-mies.

24. He anoints my head with oil!

25. My cup runs over!

26. The Lord is my shepherd!

27. I SHALL NOT WANT! (I shall not want for anything that is not already mine or available to me through the Lord Jesus!)

28. I shall not covet anything or anyone!

29. I shall not want for any good thing that is from the Lord or that is God's will that I should have!

30. Surely, goodness and mercy shall follow me all the days of my life and I will dwell in the house of the Lord forever!
31. I do some sort of stretching and exercise every day.
32. I enjoy walking the dogs and look forward to it!
33. I am the RIGHTEOUSNESS OF GOD IN CHRIST!
34. I have God's MERCY!
35. I have God's GRACE!
36. I have the POWER OF THE HOLY SPIRIT evidenced in me.
37. I lay hands on the sick in the name of Jesus, and they shall recover, in the name of Jesus!
38. I can do all things through Christ who strengthens me!
39. I have beautiful eyes.
40. I have a very nice nose.
41. My hair is growing fuller every day.
42. My body is growing stronger every day!
43. I am growing more youthful and toned and beautiful every day.
44. I do not overindulge with alcohol or other mind-numbing substances.
45. God wants me to ENJOY MY LIFE!
46. I am ALIVE with Christ!
47. I am free from the law of sin and death!
48. I will not live in fear!
49. I am born of God, and satan can't touch me.
50. I have the mind of Christ, and He leads me into His way of thinking, giving me knowledge and wisdom as each situation arises!
51. I have the peace of God that surpasses all understanding.
52. The Spirit of God, who is greater than the enemy in the world, lives in me!
53. I have received the power of the Holy Ghost and He can do miraculous things through me.
54. I have authority and power over the enemy in this world.
55. I am merciful, I do not judge others, and I forgive quickly. As I do this by God's grace, He blesses my life!

56. God supplies all my needs according to His riches in glory in Christ Jesus. He owns all the cattle on a thousand hills. I get to cash in my cattle.
57. No matter what happens, I live by faith in God.
58. I am born again—spiritually transformed, renewed, and set apart for God's purpose—through the living and eternal word of God.
59. I am God's workmanship, created in Christ to do the good works which He wants me to do!
60. I am a totally new creation, bought by the Blood of the Lamb, Jesus Christ, who gave me eternal life!

FINAL THOUGHTS AND PRAYER

Just a very important comment:

WE CANNOT BE FULLY
GRATEFUL TO GOD
IF WE DON'T OPERATE
IN GOD'S JOY, WHICH COMES WITH PEACE.
JOY IS ONE OF THE
FRUITS OF THE HOLY SPIRIT
WHICH WE RECEIVE AT SALVATION
THROUGH CHRIST JESUS,
OUR LORD AND SAVIOR!
WE ONLY HAVE TO PRAY AND SEEK
TO ACHIEVE PEACE, JOY AND CONTENTMENT.
MOMENTARILY AT FIRST,
THEN HOURLY, DAILY, WEEKLY,
MONTHLY, THEN PERMANENTLY!

Rosemary

***Help me abandon
my shameful ways;
for Your regulations are good.
I long to obey Your commandments!
Renew my life with Your goodness.***
(Psalm 119:39–40 NLT)

Oh, Father God, in the name of Jesus, please just help me with The
A.N.G.E.L. Plan©*!*

***Thank You that You are already helping me and answering
my prayers!***

Jesus, thank You that You are always just a breath away!

BIBLIOGRAPHY

Versions of the King James Holy Bible:
> Amplified Bible
> Amplified Bible Classic Edition
> English Standard Version
> 21st Century King James Version
> New King James Version
> New Living Translation
> New International Version

Merritt, Frank, and Phil White. *The 17 Hour Fast: Reset Your Eating to Revitalize Your Life*, 2018.

Mayo Clinic website at www.mayoclinic.org.

ABOUT THE AUTHOR

Rosemary Ryan-Delp is a Christian lady who has lived in many states in the country and has settled in Ozark, Arkansas. Rosemary has two sons, four daughters, topped with five grandsons and four granddaughters!

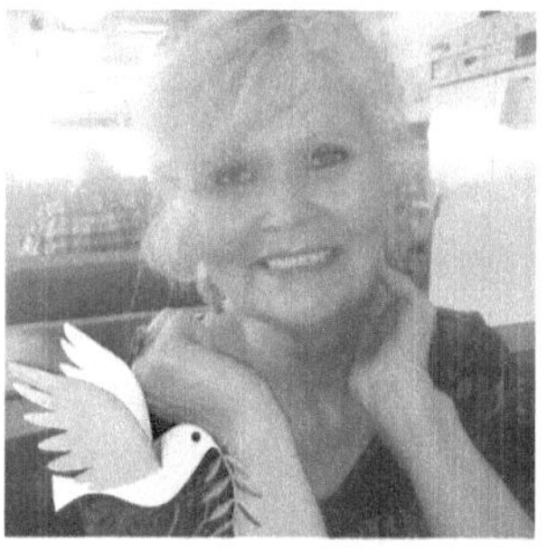

She has fought and survived a battle with food and the diet roller coaster, and has successfully incorporated *The A.N.G.E.L. Plan* into her everyday life for five years now and has won the battle with the enemy using the word of God, prayer, intermittent fasting, and lots of water. It's a unique formula that has worked for her. To God be the glory!